There's a Food
For That!

The Top 100 Foods
to fight the
Top 100 Diseases and Conditions
In the United States

By
Mark Trudeau
and
Dr Sadegh Arab

Additional copies can be obtained from your local bookstore or Amazon Publishing

www.TheresAFoodForThat.com

First Edition Copyright © 2024 Mark J. Trudeau

Manufactured in the United States of America

Library of Congress Cataloging in Publication Data
Trudeau, Mark J.
    There's a Food for That : The Top 100 Foods to fight the Top 100 Diseases and Conditions in the United States / Mark J. Trudeau and Dr. Sadegh Arab.
    Includes Index.

Disclaimer

The publisher and the author are providing this book and its contents on an "as is" basis and make no representations or warranties of any kind with respect to this book or its contents. The publisher and the author disclaim all such representations and warranties, including but not limited to warranties of healthcare for a particular purpose. In addition, the publisher and the author assume no responsibility for errors, inaccuracies, omissions, or any other inconsistencies herein.

The content of this book is for informational purposes only and is not intended to diagnose, treat, cure, or prevent any condition or disease. You understand that this book is not intended as a substitute for consultation with a licensed practitioner. Please consult with your own physician or healthcare specialist regarding the suggestions and recommendations made in this book. The use of this book implies your acceptance of this disclaimer.

The publisher and the author make no guarantees concerning the level of success you may experience by following the advice and strategies contained in this book, and you accept the risk that results will differ for each individual. The testimonials and examples provided in this book show exceptional results, which may not apply to the average reader, and are not intended to represent or guarantee that you will achieve the same or similar results.

Table of Contents

About the Authors

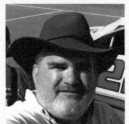

Mark Trudeau is a distinguished Data Scientist with a BS in Mathematics from Michigan Technological University and an MS in Statistics from Michigan State University. He specializes in analyzing large data sets in Manufacturing and Medical Research.

In the early 1990s, Mark co-developed the Six Sigma Black Belt Certification, collaborating with Eastman Kodak and Motorola. His expertise encompasses Designed Experiments, Data Analysis, Statistical Process Control, and Six Sigma. His ability to coach and drive continuous improvement with numerous teams has been instrumental in his contributions to this project and book.

Mark's greatest strength is his talent for presenting data in a clear and understandable manner. He excels in using optimal graphical methods and metrics to ensure that all participants can easily understand the data and results. Mark currently spends time promoting Six Sigma Black Belt Certifications while he continues to do data analysis for medical research projects, lecture, and consult.

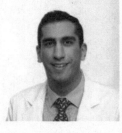

Dr. Sadegh Arab is a distinguished Doctor of Podiatric Medicine based in Michigan. He completed his undergraduate degree in Brain, Behavior, and Cognitive Sciences from the University of Michigan, which laid a solid foundation for his medical career. He then pursued his Doctorate in Podiatric Medicine at a Podiatric Medical School in Cleveland, Ohio. After completing his studies, Dr. Arab returned to Michigan to undertake a rigorous three-year residency in Podiatric Medicine and Surgery at the renowned Kern Residency Program. Currently, he practices as a podiatrist at a private practice, where he is dedicated to the comprehensive care of his patients.

Dr. Arab is a passionate advocate for preventative medicine. He strongly believes that many health issues can be prevented or managed through conscious lifestyle and dietary choices. This principle inspired him to collaborate with Mark Trudeau to write the book "There's a Food for That." Their work aims to educate readers on the benefits of a healthy diet, emphasizing the role of nutrition in disease prevention and overall wellness. Dr. Arab's commitment to patient education and preventative care is at the heart of his medical practice, where he strives to empower individuals to take control of their health.

CHAPTER 1 – Why Did We Write This Book

This journey began when I (Mark Trudeau) received the results of a blood test from our family physician, which showed for the first time that I had concerning markers: high blood sugar, high triglycerides, and elevated liver enzymes. The doctor advised me to "eat more fruits and vegetables, and avoid fast food." While avoiding fast food was straightforward, I was left wondering which specific fruits and vegetables I should include in my diet. Unfortunately, the doctor didn't have a clear answer for that.

With a background in optimizing manufacturing processes, developing algorithms, conducting medical device research and development, and other technical areas, I approached this challenge as another project to tackle. In the early 1990s, I was part of a team that developed the concept of "Six Sigma Black Belts," becoming one of the first in the industry. Thus, embarking on a project to find the best diet for my health issues felt like a natural progression.

I began researching online and quickly discovered that my blood test results were linked to Type 2 Diabetes, a condition prevalent in my family. Determined to improve my blood markers, I delved into a wealth of information, only to find inconsistencies and contradictions in the advice available. It was challenging to find consistent guidance on what foods to eat. As a data scientist, I sought precise information, wanting to know exactly which vegetables and fruits to consume instead of vague suggestions.

With the help of my friend, Dr. Sadegh Arab, we meticulously crafted a diet tailored to my needs, refining it continuously. After 36 days of following this regimen, my blood markers improved significantly, demonstrating the diet's effectiveness. This success highlighted the importance of informed dietary choices in maintaining health.

As we worked on this project, colleagues and acquaintances began seeking our help for their own health concerns, such as hypertension, diverticulitis, and multiple sclerosis. This inspired us to consider a larger initiative: analyzing data on various diseases to identify the best foods for managing each condition. With support from family, friends, coworkers, and clients, we embarked on this comprehensive project.

Initially, we had to reevaluate our approach, recognizing the need for more precise data and focusing on diseases and conditions prevalent in the United States. This led to the creation of a list, "The Top 100 Diseases and Conditions in the United States," and subsequently, "The Top 100 Foods" beneficial for these conditions. We committed to basing our recommendations on rigorous medical studies and research from reputable institutions, avoiding opinions or anecdotal advice. We worked our way through hundreds of thousands of articles and studies, ultimately compiling over 60,000 total studies on the top 100 diseases. The application of modern data science techniques allowed us to systematically analyze and summarize the wealth of information from medical journals.

After five years of dedicated work, we completed our book. Our goal is to provide readers with clear, scientifically backed dietary guidance for various diseases and conditions. Rather than offering general advice like "eat more fruits and vegetables," we provide specific recommendations, enabling people to make informed choices for their health. We hope readers find our book a valuable resource, offering direct and data-driven insights into nutrition and health.

Would You Like to Contribute?

This is our first edition, and we hope it proves to be both useful and informative. We are already planning a second edition and would greatly appreciate your feedback. If you noticed that a particular disease or condition was not included and feel it should be, or if you have suggestions for additional information, please let us know. We also welcome any corrections, including misspellings.

We value your input and, as a token of our appreciation, anyone who provides suggestions will receive a complimentary copy of our second edition upon its release. Additionally, we may acknowledge contributors in the book. Please send all suggestions to theresafoodforthat@yahoo.com. We look forward to hearing from you!

CHAPTER 2 – Scientific Method

Our study began by compiling a list of the most prevalent diseases and conditions in the United States for 2022. Prevalence was calculated based on a population of 333.3 million people, encompassing all ages and genders. Essentially, we determined the number of people affected by each disease or condition in 2022, divided that number by 333.3 million, and then multiplied by 1,000 to express prevalence per 1,000 individuals.

Chapter 3, Part 1

Top 100 Diseases and Conditions Ranked

- Research and Develop list of Top 100 Diseases and Conditions (based on the prevalence in the U.S. in 2022)
- Write a short description of each
- Do an Internet web crawl of all Medical Journals, Universities, Hospitals, and Associations that may have information on foods related (good or bad) to the Top 100 Diseases and Conditions.
- Develop Top 10 Food List for each of the 100 Top Diseases and Conditions
- Identify "Golden Bullets", defined as any food in which at least 90% of the studies listed it as a good food.
- Identify "Bad Foods", defined as any food in which at least 50% of the studies listed it as a bad food.

After creating a list of the top 100 diseases and conditions, we assembled a data science team to gather and analyze studies related to foods associated with these health issues. We paid close attention to the credibility of the studies, who conducted them, and which foods were involved. We ensured that each study was counted only once, as many were published in multiple journals, requiring careful data cleaning.

From this data, we identified the top 10 foods for each disease or condition. If a food was recommended in at least 90% of the studies, we classified it as a "Golden Bullet," indicating a strong consensus on its benefits, such as "almonds are good for gout." The remaining foods in the top 10 were labeled "Silver Bullets." For most conditions, we identified between 50 to 100 foods. Additionally, we noted if any of the top 100 foods were considered harmful for a particular condition; if at least 50% of the studies agreed, we classified the food as bad for that condition.

For the statistical calculations, it was essential to determine the standard serving sizes for all the foods. This task proved challenging, as there is often no consensus on serving sizes in the United States. Nonetheless, we devoted considerable effort to compiling this information, resulting in the table presented in Appendix 1..

Appendix 1

Serving Sizes

- Develop a table of the Standardized Serving Sizes of each of the Top 100 Foods

---

Another essential component was the table of recommended Dietary Reference Intakes (DRI) for all nutrients found in foods. We sourced this information from the National Institutes of

---

Appendix 2

Dietary Reference Intakes (DRI)

- Develop a list of the Top Nutrients found in Food
- Develop a table of the Daily Reference Intakes (DRI) of the Top Nutrients

---

Health, as indicated in the table. This data allows us to determine the nutrient content of a single serving of any given food..

With the Top 100 diseases and conditions in the United States identified, along with the Top 10 foods for each, standard serving sizes, and nutrient content, we proceeded to Chapter 4, "Top 100 Foods Ranked." We used the prevalence of each disease or condition as a weighting factor and the percentage occurrence of each food in the studies as a variable to develop a nonparametric ranking of all the foods. It's important to note that we identified

| **Chapter 4** |
| **Top 100 Foods Ranked** |
| • Using the Prevalence of each disease, develop a Nonparametric Ranking of the Top 100 Foods |
| • Collect pictures of each food from Pixabay.com |
| • Develop a table for each food, that includes all the diseases that it was listed as a top 10, identifying the Golden Bullets, and Silver Bullets |
| • Using Appendix 1, 2 (Serving Size, Daily Referance Intakes), and the USDA Website (fdc.nal.usda.gov), develop a table that lists all nutrients in each food that are at least 10% of the DRI. |

455 different foods across all articles, all of which were included in this ranking.

The outcome was a comprehensive list, ranked, of the best foods to consume for combating various diseases. After finalizing the list, we added details about the nutrients present in each food and their amounts relative to the Dietary Reference Intakes (DRI). This nutrient table aimed to answer the question, "Why do we eat this food?"

Chapter 5 builds naturally on the data we collected. In addition to identifying the Top 10 foods for each disease, we were able to create a Top 10 list of foods for each nutrient. This is

| **Chapter 5** |
| **Top 10 Foods by Nutrient** |
| • Using the Nutrient tables found in Chapter 4, rank the Top 10 Foods for each given nutrient |

particularly useful for individuals looking to increase their intake of specific nutrients, such as iron or vitamin C. By organizing our data by nutrient, we provided a clear guide to the best food sources for each nutrient.

For instance, our study revealed that yellow bell peppers contain more than three times the amount of vitamin C per serving compared to oranges, contrary to what my family previously believed. As a result, we now personally incorporate yellow bell peppers into our daily diet.

In summary, our scientific method was a significant undertaking. It took years of research to ensure the accuracy of our data, including verifying information, avoiding double counting, and correctly identifying the appropriate foods. Upon completing this process, we reviewed and summarized our scientific approach, making it clear and comprehensible. Although our book contains a substantial amount of mathematical and statistical analysis, we chose not to delve into the technical details, aiming instead for an easy-to-read and self-explanatory format.

CHAPTER 3 – Top 100 Diseases and Conditions Ranked

This table represents a significant portion of the challenge we faced while writing this book. Compiling this comprehensive list was incredibly difficult, despite how straightforward it might appear. This information is unique to our work and does not exist elsewhere. It was crucial to study every disease or condition in the United States and calculate its prevalence.

To determine prevalence, we needed to find the number of people in the United States who had each condition at any point in 2022 and then divide that number by the total U.S. population of 333.3 million in 2022. We then multiplied this figure by 1,000, as prevalence is defined by how many people out of 1,000 have a given condition. It's important to note that age and gender were not considered in this calculation. For example, even though only women can be pregnant, we still divided the number of pregnancies by 333.3 million. If the prevalence of pregnancy is 11.1, it means that 3.7 million people in the United States experienced pregnancy in 2022.

Top 100 Diseases/Conditions in USA (Ranked by Prevalence)

#	Condition	Value	#	Condition	Value	#	Condition	Value	#	Condition	Value
1	Common Cold/Virus	1000	26	Kidney Stone	88.0	51	Conjunctivitis	18.2	76	Congenital Heart Defect	7.7
2	Gastroenteritis	579.8	27	Type II Diabetes	86.0	52	ADHD	18.2	77	Celiac Disease	7.5
3	Obesity	347.3	28	Influenza	83.0	53	Menopause	17.7	78	Hypothyroidism	6.7
4	Diverticulitis	336.3	29	Asthma	76.9	54	Alzheimer's/Dementia	17.6	79	Gastritis	5.9
5	Allergies Rhinitis	300.0	30	Tinnitus	74.3	55	Bipolar Disorder	17.3	80	Type I Diabetes	5.5
6	Atopic Dermatitis	261.0	31	Cataracts	74.2	56	Iron Deficiency Anemia	15.2	81	Chlamydia	5.3
7	Insomnia	250.0	32	Sleep Apnea	66.9	57	Peptic Ulcer	13.7	82	Streptococcal Pharyngitis	5.0
8	Oral/Dental Health	239.9	33	Depression	64.3	58	Contact Dermatitis	13.6	83	Mononucleosis	5.0
9	GERD/Heartburn	230.0	34	Gallstone	60.8	59	Chronic Liver Disease,	13.4	84	Hepatitis B	4.6
10	Hypertension	228.0	35	Coronary Artery Disease	56.0	60	Inguinal Hernia	12.8	85	Autism	4.4
11	Osteoporosis	171.3	36	Arrhythmia	55.6	61	Constipation	12.1	86	Rheumatoid Arthritis	4.4
12	Alopecia Areata	170.2	37	Rosacea	48.9	62	Hyperthyroidism	12.0	87	Cancer: Colon	4.1
13	Acne	152.0	38	Endometriosis	40.0	63	Schizophrenia	12.0	88	Raynaud's Syndrome	4.0
14	Genital Herpes	152.0	39	Lumbar Radiculopathy	40.0	64	Pregnancy	11.1	89	Cancer: Skin/Melanoma	3.7
15	Chronic Kidney Disease	149.0	40	Tuberculosis	39.5	65	Epilepsy	10.8	90	HIV	3.4
16	Anxiety Disorder	141.9	41	Cold Sores	37.6	66	Cancer: Breast	10.8	91	Stroke/TIA	3.4
17	Plantar Warts	140.0	42	Fibroids	36.5	67	Hepatitis C	10.2	92	Shingles	3.0
18	Migraine	120.0	43	Hemorrhoids	30.4	68	Cancer: Prostate	9.6	93	Multiple Sclerosis	3.0
19	Urinary Tract Infection	110.0	44	Syncope	28.9	69	Inflammatory Bowel Disease	9.3	94	Parkinson's	3.0
20	High Cholesterol	102.4	45	Peripheral Arterial Disease	25.8	70	OCD	9.2	95	Cancer: Thyroid	2.5
21	Vertigo	100.0	46	Gout	25.2	71	Anemia of Chronic Disease	9.1	96	Cancer: Uterus/Endometrial	2.4
22	Premenstrual Syndrome	97.0	47	Valvular Heart Disease	25.0	72	Pneumonia	9.1	97	Cancer: Bladder	2.2
23	COPD	93.6	48	Psoriasis	24.3	73	Glaucoma	8.2	98	C: Non-Hodgkin's Lymphoma	2.2
24	Irritable Bowel Syndrome	92.9	49	Aortic Aneurysm	22.0	74	Fibromyalgia	8.2	99	Brain Tumors	2.1
25	Osteoarthritis	91.2	50	Heart Failure	19.8	75	Pelvic Inflammatory Disease	7.9	100	Cardiomyopathy	2.0

For each of the 100 diseases and conditions, the table also presents the Top 10 foods. These foods were most frequently referenced in thousands of studies conducted by various hospitals and universities over the years. If a food was consistently mentioned in at least 90% of the studies, we classified it as a "Golden Bullet," indicating broad consensus on its benefits for that condition. The other foods in the list are referred to as "Silver Bullets." The Top 10 foods are ranked in order, with the #10 food being cited frequently enough to be included in the list for that specific condition.

During the development of the list, we observed a distinction between diseases and conditions. For example, pregnancy is not a disease but a condition. This distinction became apparent during our beta testing, as people wanted guidance on what to eat for such conditions. As a result, we expanded the scope of the book from focusing solely on "Diseases" to include both "Diseases and Conditions."

In conclusion, regarding whether the recommended foods are intended for individuals who already have the disease or for those seeking to prevent it, the answer is that these foods serve both purposes. They are beneficial for prevention as well as for managing the condition if it is already present. As with any recommendations in literature of this nature, it is crucial to consult with your healthcare provider and conduct your own research (which we emphasize at the beginning). Nevertheless, these recommendations are based on robust scientific studies. For example, if someone already has Type II Diabetes, the food list provided remains applicable and useful both for managing the condition and for preventive measures. While there may be individual circumstances where certain foods might not be suitable, the recommended options represent the best choices available.

On the right, you'll find an example of a "Top 10 Foods" table, which is representative of the tables provided for each of the Top 100 Foods. In this example, the condition is Gastroenteritis. The table lists the ten most recommended foods for managing Gastroenteritis. Foods highlighted in gold are termed "Golden Bullets"; these are foods consistently identified in over 90% of studies related to the condition. The remaining foods, referred to as "Silver Bullets,"

Top 10 Foods: Gastroenteritis			
All Wild Caught/Organic/Grass-Fed/etc			
1	Apples	6	Eggs
2	Ginger Root	7	Salmon
3	Brown Rice	8	Strawberries
4	Bananas	9	Whole Oats
5	Chicken	10	Cantaloupe

Bad Foods: Gastroenteritis	
Of the Foods Included in the Top 100	
Cheese	Red Wine
Milk	Tomatoes

are also valuable but are less consistently highlighted. The list ranks these foods from most to least recommended. For instance, apples are the most frequently endorsed food, while cantaloupe, ranked 10th, is also beneficial but less prominent. This list is derived from a broader selection of 50 foods identified as beneficial for Gastroenteritis, with these ten being the top recommendations. Additionally, the table includes foods that are consistently identified as "Bad Foods" for the condition, meaning they were deemed detrimental in at least 50% of the studies. For example, cheese is considered unsuitable for Gastroenteritis.

1.   Common Cold / Virus

Prevalence: 1000 (per 1000 people in USA)

Cold and flu are both respiratory infections caused by a virus. Most medications used to treat cold/flu do not destroy or even attack the virus itself; they treat the symptoms. Our own immune system is actually the main source of our defense when it comes to preventing and fighting cold/flu viruses. Therefore, it is essential for our immune system to be optimal when cold/flu viruses are encountered. Several nutritional foods containing vitamins such as C and D, antioxidants, zinc, iron, selenium, and fiber can help strengthen our immune system. Garlic cloves are often praised for their potential immune-boosting properties, with some studies suggesting that they may help reduce the severity and duration of common cold symptoms due to their antimicrobial and anti-inflammatory compounds. Lemons, rich in vitamin C, can also be beneficial during a cold as they may support the immune system and provide relief from symptoms, such as soothing a sore throat when added to warm water or tea.

Top 10 Foods: Common Cold / Virus			
All Wild Caught/Organic/Grass-Fed/etc			
1	Garlic Cloves	6	Local Honey
2	Lemons	7	Salmon
3	Spinach	8	Apples
4	Ginger Root	9	Kale
5	Oranges	10	Broccoli

2.   Gastroenteritis

Prevalence: 579.8 (per 1000 people in USA)

Gastroenteritis is the infection and inflammation of the digestive system, mainly the intestines. Gastroenteritis can be caused by bacteria, viruses, parasites, chemicals, and at times, adverse effects from certain foods or medications. Symptoms include nausea, vomiting, abdominal pain and cramping, diarrhea, and other signs of infection such as fever and chills. During gastroenteritis, a condition characterized by inflammation of the stomach and intestines, easily digestible foods like apples and bananas can be gentle on the digestive system, providing necessary nutrients without exacerbating symptoms. Additionally, ginger root, known for its anti-nausea properties, is often recommended to help soothe the stomach and provide relief during bouts of gastroenteritis.

Top 10 Foods: Gastroenteritis			
All Wild Caught/Organic/Grass-Fed/etc			
1	Apples	6	Eggs
2	Ginger Root	7	Salmon
3	Brown Rice	8	Strawberries
4	Bananas	9	Whole Oats
5	Chicken	10	Cantaloupe

Bad Foods: Gastroenteritis	
Of the Foods Included in the Top 100	
Cheese	Red Wine
Milk	Tomatoes

3. Obesity

Prevalence: 347.3 (per 1000 people in USA)

Obesity is a very prevalent and serious problem. Obesity is defined as excessive body fat that often leads to numerous serious other health problems. Obesity often results from consuming more calories than are burned by exercise and normal daily activities. Obesity occurs when a person's body mass index is 30 or greater. Obesity has shown to have genetic correlations as well. Management of obesity is very important because of the

Top 10 Foods: Obesity			
All Wild Caught/Organic/Grass-Fed/etc			
1	Broccoli	6	Whole Oats
2	Eggs	7	Blueberries
3	Avocados	8	Greek Yogurt
4	Salmon	9	Grapefruit
5	Almonds	10	Black Beans

number of serious complications it can result in. In combating obesity, incorporating nutrient-dense foods like broccoli is crucial, as it is low in calories and high in fiber, promoting a feeling of fullness and supporting weight management. Eggs, rich in protein and essential nutrients, can also be beneficial, as they contribute to satiety and may help regulate appetite. Avocados, despite their higher calorie content, provide monounsaturated fats that promote a sense of satisfaction and can be part of a balanced diet when consumed in moderation during weight management efforts. .

4. Diverticulitis

Prevalence: 336.3 (per 1000 people in USA)

Diverticula are small bulging pouches along the lining of the intestines, more commonly in the lower part of the large intestine. Diverticulitis is a condition where these pouches become inflamed and, in some cases, infected. Diverticulitis can cause severe abdominal pain, nausea, fever, and changes in bowel movements. Diverticulitis can impact quality of life, daily activities, and performance. It should be managed properly

Top 10 Foods: Diverticulitis			
All Wild Caught/Organic/Grass-Fed/etc			
1	Apples	6	Brown Rice
2	Carrots	7	Avocados
3	Whole Wheat	8	Sweet Potatoes
4	Pears	9	Squash
5	Whole Oats	10	Potatoes

to help prevent severe outcomes and serious complications. For individuals with diverticulitis, incorporating low-fiber foods like peeled and cooked apples may be easier on the digestive system, as the removal of skins reduces fiber content, potentially alleviating symptoms. Similarly, carrots, when cooked and well-tolerated, can offer a nutrient-rich option with reduced fiber, supporting those with diverticulitis by providing essential vitamins while minimizing potential irritation to the digestive tract.

5. Allergies Rhinitis

Prevalence: 300.0 (per 1000 people in USA)

Allergic rhinitis, also known as hay fever, is an allergic response to a specific allergen,
commonly pollen. Symptoms include runny nose, sneezing, itching, coughing, hives and several other symptoms. Allergic rhinitis has a high prevalence and can vary with seasonal and geographic changes. Although Allergic Rhinitis does not usually lead to very serious

Top 10 Foods: Allergies Rhinitis			
All Wild Caught/Organic/Grass-Fed/etc			
1	Salmon	6	Ginger Root
2	Strawberries	7	Oranges
3	Onions	8	Walnuts
4	Local Honey	9	Garlic Cloves
5	Mackerel	10	Lemons

complications, it can decrease quality of life, performance, and daily activities. Proper management can help maintain quality of life. Salmon, rich in omega-3 fatty acids, has anti-inflammatory properties that may help alleviate rhinitis symptoms by modulating immune responses and reducing inflammation. Strawberries, packed with vitamin C and antioxidants, can support overall immune health, while local honey may contain trace amounts of local pollen, potentially desensitizing the immune system and offering relief for some individuals with rhinitis.

6. Atopic Dermatitis

Prevalence: 261.0 (per 1000 people in USA)

Atopic dermatitis, also known as eczema, is a very common skin condition resulting in redness and itchiness. It is commonly found in children but can exhibit symptoms in adulthood as well. Genetic correlations have been found to play a role in this condition. Atopic dermatitis can present the following: itchiness, redness, dryness, pigmented patches and bumps, scaling, swelling, and other symptoms.

Salmon, sardines, and mackerel are rich sources of omega-3 fatty acids, particularly EPA and DHA, which have anti-inflammatory properties that may benefit individuals with atopic dermatitis by reducing skin

Top 10 Foods: Atopic Dermatitis			
All Wild Caught/Organic/Grass-Fed/etc			
1	Salmon	6	Beets
2	Sardines	7	Kefir
3	Mackerel	8	Apples
4	Whole Oats	9	Walnuts
5	Herring	10	Flaxseeds

Bad Foods: Atopic Dermatitis	
Of the Foods Included in the Top 100	
Cheese	Oranges
Eggs	Soybeans
Greek Yogurt	Tomatoes
Milk	

inflammation and supporting overall skin health. The essential fatty acids found in these fatty fish can help maintain the skin's natural barrier function, potentially alleviating symptoms and contributing to the management of atopic dermatitis.

7.   Insomnia

Prevalence: 250.0 (per 1000 people in USA)

Insomnia is a sleeping disorder where a person has difficulty falling asleep, staying asleep, or both. Insomnia can vary greatly in severity. Some individuals may experience short-term insomnia caused by a stressful or traumatic event. Chronic insomnia can cause long term fatigue and lack of energy leading to mood changes, irritability, lower performance levels and overall daily function and health. Insomnia affects many individuals around the

Top 10 Foods: Insomnia			
All Wild Caught/Organic/Grass-Fed/etc			
1	Almonds	6	Brown Rice
2	Chamomile Tea	7	Walnuts
3	Salmon	8	Herring
4	Mackerel	9	Turkey
5	Whole Oats	10	Cherries

United States. Insomnia can be a primary problem, or it can be associated with other medical conditions or medications. Almonds contain magnesium, a mineral that plays a role in regulating sleep and promoting relaxation, making them a potential snack to support better sleep quality. Chamomile tea, known for its mild sedative properties, contains compounds like apigenin that can have a calming effect, potentially aiding in the management of insomnia by promoting relaxation and facilitating a more restful sleep.

8.   Oral / Dental Health

Prevalence: 239.9 (per 1000 people in USA)

Most individuals often forget about their oral health until they are reminded by their dentist. Dental health is as important as the rest of the body and can present with very serious complications if neglected. As with the rest of the body, there are certain nutrients that can help optimize one's oral health, which includes Tonsilloliths (tonsil stones). Some examples include: calcium, phosphorus, vitamin B9, vitamin C, and fiber.

Top 10 Foods: Oral / Dental Health			
All Wild Caught/Organic/Grass-Fed/etc			
1	Spinach	6	Apples
2	Kale	7	Broccoli
3	Almonds	8	Carrots
4	Greek Yogurt	9	Milk
5	Cheese	10	Garlic

A good oral/dental health can lead to a better quality of life. Spinach and kale, packed with vitamins A and C, contribute to oral health by promoting gum health and collagen production, essential for maintaining the integrity of the gums and surrounding tissues. Greek yogurt, rich in calcium and probiotics, supports strong teeth and a healthy oral microbiome, helping to prevent tooth decay and maintain overall oral hygiene.

9. GERD / Heartburn

Prevalence: 230.0 (per 1000 people in USA)

Gastroesophageal reflux disease (GERD) occurs stomach acid refluxes back into the esophagus leading to irritation. This can cause symptoms such as burning sensation around chest, difficulty swallowing, sour taste, chest pain, feeling of a lump in throat and several others. GERD can vary greatly in degree of severity among individuals. GERD occurs among many people around the United States. GERD can have a noticeable impact on daily activities, performance, and quality of life. Whole oats and brown rice, being low-acid and high-fiber foods, are gentle on the digestive system and can help alleviate symptoms of GERD by reducing stomach acid. Ginger root, known for its anti-inflammatory properties, may help soothe the digestive tract, while cantaloupe, with its low acidity and high water content, can be a hydrating and less irritating option for individuals managing GERD.

Top 10 Foods: GERD / Heartburn			
All Wild Caught/Organic/Grass-Fed/etc			
1	Whole Oats	6	Sweet Potatoes
2	Ginger Root	7	Fennel
3	Brown Rice	8	Chicken
4	Cantaloupe	9	Almonds
5	Carrots	10	Walnuts

Bad Foods: GERD / Heartburn	
Of the Foods Included in the Top 100	
Cheese	Limes
Dark Chocolate	Onions
Garlic Cloves	Oranges
Grapefruit	Tomatoes
Lemons	

10. Hypertension

Prevalence: 228.0 (per 1000 people in USA)

High blood pressure is a common disease that results in a higher than normal force that blood places on the walls of arteries, leading to heart disease. Blood pressure takes into account the amount of blood the heart pumps and the amount of resistance to blood flow in arteries. Although, there are genetic ties to having high blood pressure, several lifestyle and nutritional changes can play a major role in maintaining a normal blood pressure. Salmon is a heart-healthy choice for individuals with hypertension due to its omega-3 fatty acids, which may help lower blood pressure and reduce inflammation. Spinach, rich in potassium and magnesium, can contribute to blood pressure regulation, while pumpkin seeds, containing potassium and heart-healthy monounsaturated fats, add to a balanced diet that supports cardiovascular health and helps manage hypertension.

Top 10 Foods: Hypertension			
All Wild Caught/Organic/Grass-Fed/etc			
1	Salmon	6	Raspberries
2	Spinach	7	Pumpkin Seeds
3	Kale	8	Pistachios
4	Strawberries	9	Sunflower Seeds
5	Bananas	10	Apples

11. Osteoporosis

Prevalence: 171.3 (per 1000 people in USA)

Osteoporosis is a condition in which the quality and density of bones are reduced, resulting in weak and brittle bones, ultimately resulting in fractures. Normally, there is constant bone turnover in the body. Osteoporosis occurs when the formation of new bone does not keep up with the loss of old bone. Key nutrients to help prevent osteoporosis can include: calcium, magnesium, potassium, and vitamins C, D, K and A. Limiting sugar, salt,

Top 10 Foods: Osteoporosis			
All Wild Caught/Organic/Grass-Fed/etc			
1	Salmon	6	Sardines
2	Kale	7	Milk
3	Collard Greens	8	Cheese
4	Cabbage	9	Turnip Greens
5	Greek Yogurt	10	Spinach

and phosphorus can also aid keep healthy bones. Osteoporosis, if not managed properly, can result in serious injuries and complications. Salmon is beneficial for osteoporosis due to its high content of vitamin D and omega-3 fatty acids, which support calcium absorption and bone health. Kale and cabbage, rich in vitamin K, contribute to bone mineralization by aiding in the synthesis of proteins essential for bone strength, making them valuable additions to a diet aimed at preventing osteoporosis.

12. Alopecia Areata

Prevalence: 170.2 (per 1000 people in USA)

Alopecia Areata is a common autoimmune condition in which hair loss is occurs in patches in the scalp, eyebrows, eyelashes, face, or other parts of the body. This hair loss disorder may be unnoticeable at first but over time, bald spots are often noticeable. Alopecia Areata occurs due to the immune system attacking one's own hair follicles. This can occur in both men and women, but it is often more significant in men. Currently, there is

Top 10 Foods: Alopecia Areata			
All Wild Caught/Organic/Grass-Fed/etc			
1	Salmon	6	Eggs
2	Mackerel	7	Almonds
3	Sardines	8	Walnuts
4	Spinach	9	Turkey
5	Chicken	10	Broccoli

no cure for Alopecia Areata. Salmon, mackerel, and sardines are excellent sources of omega-3 fatty acids, which possess anti-inflammatory properties that may potentially benefit individuals with alopecia areata by modulating the immune response and reducing inflammation around hair follicles. These fatty fish also provide essential nutrients like vitamin D and protein, supporting overall scalp health and potentially contributing to hair growth in those affected by alopecia areata.

13. Acne

Prevalence: 152.0 (per 1000 people in USA)

Acne is a skin condition characterized by the formation of pimples, blackheads, and whiteheads, often resulting from the clogging of hair follicles with oil and dead skin cells. Hormonal changes, excess oil production, and bacteria contribute to the development of acne, which commonly appears on the face, chest, and back. It can range from mild to severe, requiring different treatment strategies for effective management. Salmon, rich in omega-3 fatty acids, may help reduce inflammation associated with acne, promoting a healthier complexion. Spinach, abundant in vitamins A and C, contributes to skin health by supporting collagen production and providing antioxidants that combat free radicals. Almonds, with their vitamin E content, can aid in protecting the skin from oxidative stress, potentially benefiting individuals with acne by promoting clearer and healthier skin. .

Top 10 Foods: Acne			
All Wild Caught/Organic/Grass-Fed/etc			
1	Salmon	6	Blueberries
2	Spinach	7	Carrots
3	Kale	8	Collard Greens
4	Almonds	9	Swiss Chard
5	Mackerel	10	Grass-Fed Beef

Bad Foods: Acne
Of the Foods Included in the Top 100
Dark Chocolate

14. Genital Herpes

Prevalence: 152.0 (per 1000 people in USA)

Genital herpes is a common sexually transmitted disease caused by the herpes simplex virus (HSV). It can be spread through sexual contact at any age or sex. The virus can remain dormant in the body after the initial infection and reactivate several times a year. Genital herpes can cause pain, itching and sores in the genital area of both males and females. Often times genital herpes can exhibit no symptoms, however, it can still be transmitted through sexual contact. Salmon and mackerel, rich in omega-3 fatty acids and lysine, may have anti-inflammatory and immune-boosting properties that could potentially aid in managing genital herpes outbreaks. Apples, containing quercetin, an antioxidant with antiviral properties, might contribute to immune system support, potentially assisting in the prevention or reduction of genital herpes symptoms.

Top 10 Foods: Genital Herpes			
All Wild Caught/Organic/Grass-Fed/etc			
1	Salmon	6	Cheese
2	Mackerel	7	Bell Peppers
3	Apples	8	Pears
4	Chicken	9	Apricots
5	Greek Yogurt	10	Mangoes

Bad Foods: Genital Herpes	
Of the Foods Included in the Top 100	
Dark Chocolate	Whole Wheat

15. Chronic Kidney Disease

Prevalence: 149.0 (per 1000 people in USA)

Chronic kidney disease, also known as chronic kidney failure, is a gradual loss of kidney function leading to serious symptoms and need for dialysis or kidney transplant. Symptoms include: nausea, vomiting, loss of appetite, fatigue, swelling, high blood pressure, chest pain, shortness of breath, and many other symptoms. Chronic kidney disease can eventually lead to End Stage Renal Disease which is a fatal condition without dialysis or kidney transplant. Chronic kidney disease is common amongst many and can affect almost every part of the body. Egg whites, being low in phosphorus, can be a beneficial

Top 10 Foods: Chronic Kidney Disease			
All Wild Caught/Organic/Grass-Fed/etc			
1	Egg Whites	6	Salmon
2	Blueberries	7	Apples
3	Bell Peppers	8	Mackerel
4	Cabbage	9	Strawberries
5	Cranberries	10	Garlic Cloves

Bad Foods: Chronic Kidney Disease	
Of the Foods Included in the Top 100	
Avocados	Potatoes
Bananas	Prunes
Oranges	

protein source for individuals with chronic kidney disease (CKD) as high phosphorus levels can be problematic for kidney function. Blueberries and bell peppers, rich in antioxidants and low in potassium, provide a nutrient-dense option for those with CKD, potentially supporting overall health and mitigating the risk of complications associated with kidney disease.

16. Anxiety Disorder

Prevalence: 141.9 (per 1000 people in USA)

Anxiety disorder presents itself with intense, excessive and persistent worry and fear about normal day to day activities. Often times, anxiety disorders involve repeated episodes of sudden feelings of intense anxiety and fear or terror that reach a peak within minutes, leading to panic attacks. People with anxiety disorder often have difficulty performing their daily activities and tend to avoid situations that can induce their symptoms.

Top 10 Foods: Anxiety Disorder			
All Wild Caught/Organic/Grass-Fed/etc			
1	Dark Chocolate	6	Chia Seeds
2	Almonds	7	Salmon
3	Whole Oats	8	Spinach
4	Eggs	9	Walnuts
5	Blueberries	10	Greek Yogurt

Multiple types of anxiety disorders exist with a wide spectrum of severity and symptoms. Dark chocolate, containing flavonoids, may contribute to anxiety reduction by promoting relaxation and improving mood through the release of endorphins. Almonds, rich in magnesium and vitamin E, can be beneficial for anxiety as these nutrients play a role in stress management and overall brain health. Whole oats, with their complex carbohydrates, may contribute to stable blood sugar levels, providing a sustained release of energy that can positively impact mood and help alleviate anxiety symptoms.

17. Plantar Warts

Prevalence: 140.0 (per 1000 people in USA)

Plantar warts are small skin lesions cause by Human Papilloma Virus (HPV) that usually appear on the heels or other weight-bearing surfaces of the feet. They often present with callus formation and can painful, have pinpoint bleeding, and produce an unattractive appearance. Although not easily transmissible, they can spread from person to person through direct contact. Although most often seen in children and teenagers, plantar

Top 10 Foods: Plantar Warts			
All Wild Caught/Organic/Grass-Fed/etc			
1	Spinach	6	Garlic Cloves
2	Oranges	7	Carrots
3	Apples	8	Avocados
4	Broccoli	9	Squash
5	Strawberries	10	Kale

warts can appear at any age. Despite rarity of any serious complication, proper management and treatment of plantar warts is warranted. A robust immune system is crucial for combating viral infections, and including proper foods in the diet may support the body's ability to naturally address plantar warts caused by the human papillomavirus (HPV).

18. Migraine

Prevalence: 120.0 (per 1000 people in USA)

Migraine headaches usually present as severe throbbing pain or a pulsing sensation, usually on one side of the head. Migraine is often accompanied by nausea, vomiting, and extreme sensitivity to light and sound. Migraine attacks can last for hours to days. Symptoms of Migraine can be so severe that they interfere with daily activities and tend to lead to mood changes, reduced performance, fatigue, and significant decrease in quality of life. Proper management of migraine is critical. Salmon, rich in omega-3 fatty acids, has anti-inflammatory properties that may help reduce the frequency and severity of migraines by mitigating inflammation in the brain. Spinach and kale, abundant in

Top 10 Foods: Migraine			
All Wild Caught/Organic/Grass-Fed/etc			
1	Salmon	6	Carrots
2	Spinach	7	Herring
3	Kale	8	Sweet Potatoes
4	Mackerel	9	Sardines
5	Chicken	10	Swiss Chard

Bad Foods: Migraine	
Of the Foods Included in the Top 100	
Cheese	Limes
Dark Chocolate	Milk
Eggs	Onions
Grapefruit	Oranges
Greek Yogurt	Red Wine
Lemons	Sauerkraut

magnesium, may contribute to migraine prevention as magnesium deficiency has been associated with an increased susceptibility to these headaches, and maintaining adequate levels of magnesium can have a positive impact on neurological function.

19. Urinary Tract Infection

Prevalence: 110.0 (per 1000 people in USA)

A urinary tract infection (UTI) is an infection in any part of your urinary system, most commonly occurring in the bladder and the urethra. Women are at a higher risk of developing UTIs as compared to men. Symptoms include: urge to urinate frequently, burning and discomfort while urinating, cloudy appearance or sometimes blood in urine, discharge, malodor or strong odor urine, and several other symptoms. It is

Top 10 Foods: Urinary Tract Infection			
All Wild Caught/Organic/Grass-Fed/etc			
1	Greek Yogurt	6	Mackerel
2	Cranberries	7	Chicken
3	Garlic Cloves	8	Strawberries
4	Kefir	9	Whole Oats
5	Salmon	10	Blueberries

important to determine the level of UTI in the urinary system to correctly treat the condition. Greek yogurt contains probiotics that may help maintain a healthy balance of bacteria in the gut, potentially preventing the spread of harmful bacteria to the urinary tract and reducing the risk of urinary tract infections (UTIs). Cranberries, known for their anti-adhesive properties, may help prevent bacteria, particularly E. coli, from adhering to the urinary tract lining, lowering the likelihood of UTIs, while garlic's antimicrobial properties may contribute to overall urinary tract health by inhibiting the growth of bacteria.

20. High Cholesterol (Hyperlipidemia)

Prevalence: 102.4 (per 1000 people in USA)

High cholesterol simply means abnormally high amounts of lipids (fats) in the bloodstream. High cholesterol can lead to many life-threatening conditions such as heart disease and stroke. Without going into too much detail regarding differences in types of lipids, LDL and triglycerides are what need to be avoided and lowered. Additionally, foods high in fiber, omega-3 fatty acids, and whey protein have shown to help lower cholesterol. A proper diet is essential in managing high cholesterol. Salmon, rich in omega-3 fatty acids, can help lower triglycerides and

Top 10 Foods: High Cholesterol			
All Wild Caught/Organic/Grass-Fed/etc			
1	Salmon	6	Strawberries
2	Almonds	7	Walnuts
3	Whole Oats	8	Avocados
4	Apples	9	Extra Virgin Olive Oil
5	Mackerel	10	Kidney Beans

reduce inflammation, contributing to improved cholesterol levels. Almonds, with their monounsaturated fats and fiber, may assist in lowering LDL (bad) cholesterol, while whole oats, containing beta-glucans, have been shown to help lower cholesterol levels, supporting cardiovascular health when incorporated into a balanced diet.

21. Vertigo

Prevalence: 100.0 (per 1000 people in USA)

Vertigo is a common medical condition where a person feels that they are in motion or objects around them are in motion when they are not. Vertigo can have several different causes. Symptoms associated with vertigo include motion sickness, nausea, vomiting, headache, and unsteady gait pattern. Patients with vertigo should be evaluated for the underlying cause of their symptoms. Vertigo can interfere with daily activities, reduce performance, and significantly decrease quality of life.

Ginger root has anti-inflammatory and anti-nausea properties that may provide relief for

Top 10 Foods: Vertigo			
All Wild Caught/Organic/Grass-Fed/etc			
1	Ginger Root	6	
2	Ginkgo Biloba	7	
3	Salmon	8	
4	Extra Virgin Olive Oil	9	
5		10	

Bad Foods: Vertigo	
Of the Foods Included in the Top 100	
Cheese	Limes
Grapefruit	Oranges
Lemons	

vertigo symptoms by reducing inflammation and calming the digestive system. Ginkgo biloba, known for its potential to enhance blood circulation, may aid in improving blood flow to the brain, potentially alleviating symptoms of vertigo associated with compromised circulation.

22. Premenstrual Syndrome

Prevalence: 97.0 (per 1000 people in USA)

Premenstrual Syndrome (PMS) is a common finding amongst women that presents itself with a variety of symptoms that tend to recur in a predictable pattern. These symptoms often include: mood swings, headache, tender breasts, abdominal bloating, food cravings, poor concentration, fatigue, irritability, Acne flare-ups, depression, and many more. The physical and emotional impacts of PMS can often interfere with daily

Top 10 Foods: Premenstrual Syndrome			
All Wild Caught/Organic/Grass-Fed/etc			
1	Salmon	6	Spinach
2	Greek Yogurt	7	Kale
3	Sardines	8	Mackerel
4	Milk	9	Broccoli
5	Peanuts	10	Almonds

activity and performance. Salmon and sardines, high in omega-3 fatty acids, may help mitigate premenstrual syndrome (PMS) symptoms by reducing inflammation and supporting hormonal balance. Greek yogurt, rich in calcium and probiotics, can contribute to PMS relief as calcium is associated with mood regulation, and the probiotics support digestive health, potentially positively impacting overall well-being during the menstrual cycle.

23. COPD

Prevalence: 93.6 (per 1000 people in USA)

Chronic obstructive pulmonary disease (COPD) is a chronic inflammatory lung condition that leads to obstruction of airflow from the lungs. Symptoms include shortness of breath, cough, mucus formation, and wheezing. COPD is normally caused by long-term exposure to irritating gases or particulate matter, most often from cigarette smoke. Emphysema and chronic bronchitis are the two most common conditions that contribute to COPD and can vary in severity. People with COPD are at higher risk of developing very serious heart and lung conditions. Salmon, rich in omega-3 fatty acids, may have anti-inflammatory effects that can benefit individuals with chronic obstructive pulmonary disease (COPD) by reducing inflammation in the airways. Oranges and carrots, high in antioxidants like vitamin C and beta-carotene, respectively, contribute to respiratory health and may help protect against oxidative stress, potentially supporting lung function in those with COPD.

Top 10 Foods: COPD			
All Wild Caught/Organic/Grass-Fed/etc			
1	Salmon	6	Squash
2	Mackerel	7	Spinach
3	Oranges	8	Kale
4	Carrots	9	Chicken
5	Grapefruit	10	Whole Oats

Bad Foods: COPD	
Of the Foods Included in the Top 100	
Barley	Greek Yogurt
Broccoli	Lentils
Brussel Sprouts	Milk
Cabbage	Onions
Cauliflower	Whole Wheat
Cheese	

24. Irritable Bowel Syndrome

Prevalence: 92.9 (per 1000 people in USA)

Irritable bowel syndrome (IBS) is a high prevalence and often chronic condition that affects the large intestine. Signs and symptoms include cramping, abdominal pain, bloating, gas, and diarrhea or constipation, or both. Most people can manage their symptoms with diet, healthy lifestyle, and by managing stress. However, a small group can develop severe symptoms, which can often be treated with medications and counseling. Symptoms from IBS, if not managed, can impact one's quality of life. Salmon, chicken, and eggs are valuable protein sources that may be well-tolerated by individuals with irritable bowel syndrome (IBS), providing essential nutrients without exacerbating digestive symptoms. Additionally, these foods are generally lower in fermentable carbohydrates, potentially reducing the risk of triggering IBS symptoms and supporting digestive comfort.

Top 10 Foods: IBS			
All Wild Caught/Organic/Grass-Fed/etc			
1	Salmon	6	Sardines
2	Mackerel	7	Eggplant
3	Chicken	8	Strawberries
4	Eggs	9	Carrots
5	Herring	10	Sweet Potatoes

25. Osteoarthritis

Prevalence: 91.2 (per 1000 people in USA)

Osteoarthritis is the a common condition that often occurs due to natural wear and tear of joints, musculoskeletal/joint injuries, age, or history of musculoskeletal/joint surgeries.

Symptoms from Osteoarthritis arise due to loss of cartilage that provides a natural cushion in the joints. Osteoarthritis can occur in any joint. Associated symptoms include: pain, stiffness, tenderness, inflexibility, spur sensation, and swelling. Patients with severe

Top 10 Foods: Osteoarthritis			
All Wild Caught/Organic/Grass-Fed/etc			
1	Salmon	6	Broccoli
2	Spinach	7	Extra Virgin Olive Oil
3	Walnuts	8	Collard Greens
4	Kale	9	Swiss Chard
5	Mackerel	10	Almonds

Osteoarthritis often opt for joint replacement or joint fusion surgeries to improve symptoms and functionality. Salmon, rich in omega-3 fatty acids, may help alleviate symptoms of osteoarthritis by reducing inflammation and supporting joint health. Spinach and walnuts, containing antioxidants and anti-inflammatory compounds, contribute to overall joint well-being, potentially providing relief for individuals with osteoarthritis by supporting the management of inflammation and maintaining joint function.

26. Kidney Stone

Prevalence: 88.0 (per 1000 people in USA)

Kidney stones are hard deposits made of minerals and salts that form inside the kidneys. Kidney stones can be caused by diet, excess body weight, certain medical conditions, and

some supplements and medications. Signs and symptoms can include: sharp and radiating pain, burning and painful urination, discharge, malodor urine, discolored urine, nausea, vomiting, fever, chills, and several others. Although many stones can pass

Top 10 Foods: Kidney Stone			
All Wild Caught/Organic/Grass-Fed/etc			
1	Kale	6	Avocados
2	Broccoli	7	Bananas
3	Chicken	8	Quinoa
4	Brown Rice	9	Turkey
5	Carrots	10	Bell Peppers

without severe outcomes, kidney stones can become a serious health risk and may need immediate medical attention. Kale, being low in oxalates, chicken, a good source of lean protein, and brown rice, a low-oxalate whole grain, are suitable choices for individuals prone to kidney stones as they may help minimize the risk of oxalate-based stone formation. Additionally, the combination of these foods contributes to a balanced diet that supports overall kidney health by providing essential nutrients while minimizing dietary factors associated with kidney stone formation.

27. Type II Diabetes

Prevalence: 86.0 (per 1000 people in USA)

Type II diabetes is a chronic condition that influences the way the body metabolizes glucose, often resulting in abnormally high blood glucose levels. Type II diabetes can be a deadly disease and needs to be taken seriously. It develops when insulin receptors, which are responsible for glucose uptake in the bloodstream, become resistant due to over stimulation caused by high carbohydrate diets. Aside from lowering carbohydrate

Top 10 Foods: Type II Diabetes			
All Wild Caught/Organic/Grass-Fed/etc			
1	Walnuts	6	Broccoli
2	Greek Yogurt	7	Strawberries
3	Salmon	8	Whole Oats
4	Spinach	9	Blueberries
5	Mackerel	10	Oranges

intake, several other dietary changes can help prevent type II diabetes. Antioxidants, vitamins, omega-3 fatty acids, and high protein diet have shown to play a major role. Walnuts, rich in omega-3 fatty acids and antioxidants, may benefit individuals with type 2 diabetes by potentially improving insulin sensitivity and managing inflammation. Greek yogurt, with its high protein content and probiotics, can contribute to blood sugar control, while salmon, being a source of lean protein and omega-3s, may support cardiovascular health, which is particularly important for individuals with type 2 diabetes who are at a higher risk of heart-related complications.

28. Influenza

Prevalence: 83.0 (per 1000 people in USA)

Cold and flu are both respiratory infections caused by a virus. Most medications used to treat cold/flu do not destroy or even attack the virus itself; they treat the symptoms. Our own immune system is actually the main source of our defense when it comes to preventing and fighting cold/flu viruses. Therefore, it is essential for our immune system to be optimal when cold/flu viruses are encountered. Several nutritional foods

Top 10 Foods: Influenza			
All Wild Caught/Organic/Grass-Fed/etc			
1	Lemons	6	Broccoli
2	Bell Peppers	7	Almonds
3	Green Tea	8	Ginger Root
4	Salmon	9	Blueberries
5	Kale	10	Oranges

containing vitamins such as C and D, antioxidants, zinc, iron, selenium, and fiber can help strengthen our immune system.

Lemons, with their high vitamin C content, bell peppers, rich in antioxidants like vitamin C and beta-carotene, and green tea, known for its immune-boosting properties, are beneficial for influenza by supporting the immune system and providing anti-inflammatory effects. These foods contribute essential nutrients and compounds that may aid in reducing the severity and duration of flu symptoms, promoting overall recovery and well-being.

29. Asthma

Prevalence: 76.9 (per 1000 people in USA)

Asthma is a very common condition that is a result of narrowing and swelling in the airways leading to wheezing, shortness of breath, mucus formation, coughing, and difficulty breathing. Asthma can occur at any age and affects both men and women. Although many can manage their Asthma without much disturbance, some can have severe Asthma attacks that can be life-threatening. There is no cure for Asthma, but symptoms

Top 10 Foods: Asthma			
All Wild Caught/Organic/Grass-Fed/etc			
1	Spinach	6	Salmon
2	Kale	7	Broccoli
3	Apples	8	Flaxseeds
4	Carrots	9	Milk
5	Sweet Potatoes	10	Sunflower Seeds

can be managed to prevent impact on quality of life and normal day to day activities. Spinach and kale, being rich in vitamins C and K, along with apples, which contain antioxidants and fiber, can be beneficial for individuals with asthma by supporting lung health and reducing inflammation. These nutrient-dense foods may contribute to improved respiratory function and overall well-being, potentially helping manage symptoms associated with asthma.

30. Tinnitus

Prevalence: 74.3 (per 1000 people in USA)

Tinnitus is normally considered a symptom of an underlying condition that results in ringing or perception of noise in the ears. Tinnitus can have many causes and a large spectrum of severity. It is important to determine the underlying cause of Tinnitus. Associated signs and symptoms that can present with Tinnitus include: Fatigue, stress, sleep problems, trouble concentrating, memory problems, depression, anxiety and irritability. Tinnitus, if

Top 10 Foods: Tinnitus			
All Wild Caught/Organic/Grass-Fed/etc			
1	Spinach	6	Chicken
2	Bananas	7	Almonds
3	Pineapple	8	Ginger Root
4	Kale	9	Walnuts
5	Broccoli	10	Avocados

left untreated, can often times affect one's quality of life. Spinach, bananas, and pineapple are rich in nutrients such as magnesium, potassium, and antioxidants, which may help improve blood circulation and reduce inflammation, potentially alleviating symptoms associated with tinnitus. Including these foods in the diet can contribute to overall ear health and may have a positive impact on managing tinnitus-related discomfort.

31. Cataracts

Prevalence: 74.2 (per 1000 people in USA)

Cataracts is the clouding of the normally clear lens of your eye. People often describe their vision as seeing through cloudy lenses, looking through a frosty or fogged-up window.

Clouded vision caused by cataracts can impede normal daily activity such as reading, driving, and facial recognition. Cataract tends to develop overtime, often being mild early on and gaining severity over time. It is important to be attentive to signs and

Top 10 Foods: Cataracts			
All Wild Caught/Organic/Grass-Fed/etc			
1	Salmon	6	Strawberries
2	Spinach	7	Almonds
3	Carrots	8	Oranges
4	Bell Peppers	9	Tomatoes
5	Broccoli	10	Grapefruit

symptoms of cataracts to prevent severe outcomes. Salmon, packed with omega-3 fatty acids, spinach, rich in antioxidants like lutein and zeaxanthin, and carrots, a source of beta-carotene, contribute to eye health and may be beneficial for preventing or slowing the progression of cataracts. These nutrients help protect the eyes from oxidative stress and support the maintenance of clear lenses, potentially reducing the risk of developing cataracts over time.

32. Sleep Apnea

Prevalence: 66.9 (per 1000 people in USA)

Sleep Apnea is a common sleeping disorder that presents as repeated stopping and starting of breathing during sleep. There are three types of sleep apnea: obstructive sleep apnea, central sleep apnea, and complex sleep apnea syndrome. Although many have mild symptoms, sleep apnea can become a serious issue and requires medical attention. Sleep apnea often affects the quality of life, daily performance, and concentration. Men are

Top 10 Foods: Sleep Apnea			
All Wild Caught/Organic/Grass-Fed/etc			
1	Cherries	6	Whole Oats
2	Salmon	7	Walnuts
3	Apples	8	Sweet Potatoes
4	Kale	9	Tomatoes
5	Broccoli	10	Milk

more frequently affected by sleep apnea than women. Sleep apnea can lead to many other serious conditions. Cherries, containing melatonin and antioxidants, may support sleep regulation and reduce inflammation, potentially benefiting individuals with sleep apnea. Salmon, rich in omega-3 fatty acids, and apples, with their natural sugars and fiber, contribute to a balanced diet that promotes overall health, potentially positively influencing sleep patterns and mitigating sleep apnea symptoms.

33. Depression

Prevalence: 64.3 (per 1000 people in USA)

Major Depressive Disorder (Depression) is a common mood disorder that causes a persistent feeling of sadness and loss of interest. Depression can have a significant impact on one's quality of life, performance, and daily activities. Depression can lead to mental and physical symptoms. Severity often varies with Depression and it is important to be managed properly. Depression can have many different causes and associations.

Top 10 Foods: Depression			
All Wild Caught/Organic/Grass-Fed/etc			
1	Avocados	6	Flaxseeds
2	Salmon	7	Chia Seeds
3	Spinach	8	Mackerel
4	Walnuts	9	Blueberries
5	Greek Yogurt	10	Herring

Depression can appear at any age and can affect both men and women. Avocados, salmon, and spinach are rich in nutrients such as omega-3 fatty acids, vitamins B, and folate, which are associated with brain health and neurotransmitter function. Including these foods in the diet may provide essential elements that support mental well-being, potentially contributing to the management of depression symptoms.

34. Gallstone

Prevalence: 60.8 (per 1000 people in USA)

Gallstones are hardened deposits of digestive fluid, varying in size, that can form in the gallbladder. One can develop single or multiple gallstones at the same time. Severity varies based on size and number of stones. Signs and symptoms include: sharp, severe, radiating pain to the right upper abdominal quadrant, nausea, vomiting, pain in shoulder, and several others. Females have a higher tendency to get gallstones than men.

Top 10 Foods: Gallstone			
All Wild Caught/Organic/Grass-Fed/etc			
1	Spinach	6	Flaxseeds
2	Kale	7	Lentils
3	Oranges	8	Salmon
4	Lemons	9	Mackerel
5	Grapefruit	10	Walnuts

Although common, gallstones can have serious complications and may require serious medical attention. Spinach, oranges, and flaxseeds can be beneficial for gallstones due to their high fiber content. Fiber helps regulate bile production and flow, potentially reducing the risk of gallstone formation by promoting efficient digestion and preventing the stagnation of bile in the gallbladder.

35. Coronary Artery Disease

Prevalence: 56.0 (per 1000 people in USA)

Coronary Artery Disease (CAD) is a common but very serious medical condition in which major arteries that supply the heart become damaged, diseased, narrowed, or obstructed, leading to decreased blood flow, and therefore, nutrients and oxygen to the heart. Common signs and symptoms start as chest pain (angina) and shortness of breath, and frequently lead to a heart attacks when a complete blockage occurs. CAD is a very

Top 10 Foods: Coronary Artery Disease			
All Wild Caught/Organic/Grass-Fed/etc			
1	Salmon	6	Walnuts
2	Mackerel	7	Herring
3	Almonds	8	Black Beans
4	Blueberries	9	Kale
5	Oranges	10	Broccoli

serious problem in the United States and has lead to many deaths. Proper management of CAD is crucial to prevent serious outcomes. Salmon, rich in omega-3 fatty acids, may contribute to cardiovascular health by reducing inflammation and supporting healthy cholesterol levels, potentially benefiting individuals with coronary artery disease. Almonds, with their monounsaturated fats and antioxidants, and blueberries, containing anthocyanins, can further support heart health by promoting lower blood pressure and reducing oxidative stress, offering potential protective effects against coronary artery disease.

36. Arrhythmia / AFib

Prevalence: 55.6 (per 1000 people in USA)

Arrhythmia is a common heart condition where the heart can beat at an abnormal pace, rhythm, or both. Arrhythmias can vary greatly in severity that can be harmless or life-threatening. It is crucial to find the underlying cause of Arrhythmia and allow proper management. Several types of Arrhythmias include atrial fibrillation (AFib), ventricular fibrillation, ventricular tachycardia, atrial flutter, and many others. Heart Arrhythmia

Top 10 Foods: Arrhythmia / Afib			
All Wild Caught/Organic/Grass-Fed/etc			
1	Salmon	6	Walnuts
2	Mackerel	7	Herring
3	Almonds	8	Black Beans
4	Blueberries	9	Kale
5	Oranges	10	Broccoli

should not be taken lightly at any age or sex. Salmon, high in omega-3 fatty acids, may have anti-arrhythmic effects, potentially reducing the risk of abnormal heart rhythms. Almonds, rich in magnesium, and blueberries, containing anthocyanins, contribute to heart health by supporting proper electrical conduction and offering antioxidant properties, which may be beneficial in managing arrhythmia.

37. Rosacea

Prevalence: 48.9 (per 1000 people in USA)

Rosacea is a common skin condition that causes redness and visible blood vessels in the face. It may also produce small, red, pus-filled bumps that can often be mistaken for Acne.

These signs and symptoms may flare up for weeks to months and present periodically and unpredictably. Rosacea can affect anyone. But it is commonly seen middle-aged women with a light skin tone. There is no cure for rosacea, but treatment can help control and reduce the signs and symptoms. Chia seeds, barley, and salmon are beneficial for individuals with rosacea due to their anti-inflammatory properties. These foods, rich in

Top 10 Foods: Rosacea			
All Wild Caught/Organic/Grass-Fed/etc			
1	Chia Seeds	6	Flaxseeds
2	Barley	7	Onions
3	Salmon	8	Asparagus
4	Whole Oats	9	Amaranth
5	Walnuts	10	Spinach

Bad Foods: Rosacea	
Of the Foods Included in the Top 100	
Dark Chocolate	Limes
Grapefruit	Oranges
Lemons	Red Wine

omega-3 fatty acids, antioxidants, and anti-inflammatory compounds, may help manage inflammation associated with rosacea and promote skin health.

38. Endometriosis

Prevalence: 40.0 (per 1000 people in USA)

Endometriosis is a common condition amongst women that can have range of symptoms with varying severities. Endometriosis is commonly defined as growth of, what is a natural

lining tissue of the uterus, outside of the uterus. This tissue thickens overtimes and sheds as it does in the uterus, however, there is no route of exit with each menstrual cycle and becomes trapped. Pain and discomfort are often times the most common complaint of endometriosis, however, others associated symptoms such as infertility can be a major problem. Salmon, high in omega-3 fatty acids,

Top 10 Foods: Endometriosis			
All Wild Caught/Organic/Grass-Fed/etc			
1	Salmon	6	Walnuts
2	Mackerel	7	Herring
3	Spinach	8	Chia Seeds
4	Kale	9	Broccoli
5	Almonds	10	Strawberries

Bad Foods: Endometriosis	
Of the Foods Included in the Top 100	
Red Wine	

spinach, rich in iron and antioxidants, and almonds, containing vitamin E and fiber, may be beneficial for individuals with endometriosis. These foods possess anti-inflammatory properties, support hormonal balance, and contribute to overall well-being, potentially assisting in managing symptoms associated with endometriosis.

39. Lumbar Radiculopathy

Prevalence: 40.0 (per 1000 people in USA)

Lumbar radiculopathy is defined as compression, inflammation, damage/injury to the spinal nerve root at the level of the lumbar spine. Signs and symptoms can not only affect the

back but can radiate to other regions and produce varying symptoms with a wide range of severity. Lumbar radiculopathy can have a wide variety of causes and affects a large population of people around the United States. Proper management is very important

Top 10 Foods: Lumbar Radiculopathy			
All Wild Caught/Organic/Grass-Fed/etc			
1	Spinach	6	Salmon
2	Kale	7	Cheese
3	Broccoli	8	Whole Oats
4	Greek Yogurt	9	Walnuts
5	Milk	10	Flaxseeds

or it can interfere with daily activities, reduce performance, and significantly decrease quality of life. Spinach and broccoli, rich in vitamins C and K, along with milk, a good source of calcium and vitamin D, can be beneficial for individuals with lumbar radiculopathy. These nutrients support bone health and may contribute to the alleviation of symptoms associated with lumbar radiculopathy by promoting spinal strength and reducing the risk of complications related to bone density.

40. Tuberculosis

Prevalence: 39.5 (per 1000 people in USA)

Tuberculosis (TB) is a medical condition affecting the lungs caused by infection by Mycobacterium tuberculosis. TB can be highly contagious through respiratory droplets.

Signs and symptoms include cough, chest pain, shortness of breath, fatigue, fever, chills, coughing up blood, and many others. TB can be in an active phase or become latent in the body. TB can cause serious manifestations, especially in

Top 10 Foods: Tuberculosis (TB)			
All Wild Caught/Organic/Grass-Fed/etc			
1	Carrots	6	Mackerel
2	Tomatoes	7	Blueberries
3	Salmon	8	Brown Rice
4	Oranges	9	Herring
5	Whole Wheat	10	Sweet Potatoes

immunocompromised individuals. TB interfere with daily activities, reduce performance, and significantly decrease quality of life. Carrots, rich in beta-carotene, tomatoes, abundant in antioxidants like lycopene, and salmon, high in omega-3 fatty acids, contribute to a nutrient-rich diet that may support overall immune function and respiratory health, which can be particularly beneficial for individuals with tuberculosis. Including these foods may provide essential vitamins and compounds that help the body combat infections and promote recovery from tuberculosis.

41. Cold Sores

Prevalence: 37.6 (per 1000 people in USA)

Cold sores are small, fluid filled blisters that form around the mouth that are caused by human herpes virus type 1 and 2 (HSV-1 & HSV-2). Cold sores can be passed from person to person by close contact. Cold sores tend to resolve quickly and can easily be managed. They can at times produce associated symptoms such as fever, sore throat, headache, swollen lymph nodes, and few others. Although often not a life-threatening condition, it can have serious manifestations in immunocompromised individuals. Salmon and mackerel, rich in omega-3 fatty acids,

Top 10 Foods: Cold Sores		
All Wild Caught/Organic/Grass-Fed/etc		
1 Salmon	6	Chicken
2 Mackerel	7	Greek Yogurt
3 Herring	8	Cheese
4 Sardines	9	Bell Peppers
5 Apples	10	Pears
Bad Foods: Cold Sores		
Of the Foods Included in the Top 100		
Dark Chocolate		Whole Wheat

may have anti-inflammatory effects that can potentially aid in the management of cold sores by reducing inflammation and supporting the immune system. Apples and chicken, containing lysine, an amino acid known to inhibit the replication of the herpes simplex virus, may contribute to the prevention and alleviation of cold sore outbreaks.

42. Fibroids

Prevalence: 36.5 (per 1000 people in USA)

Fibroids are benign tissue growths, varying in size and number, that happen in women's uterus. They can often present without symptoms and go unnoticed or only come to attention as an incidental finding. If symptomatic, signs include: heavy menstrual bleeding, menstrual periods lasting more than a week, pelvic pressure or pain, frequent urination, difficulty emptying the bladder, constipation, backache, or leg pains. Although benign, fibroids can affect quality of life and daily activities. Broccoli and collard greens, being cruciferous vegetables, contain

Top 10 Foods: Fibroids		
All Wild Caught/Organic/Grass-Fed/etc		
1 Broccoli	6	Kale
2 Collard Greens	7	Whole Oats
3 Cabbage	8	Carrots
4 Salmon	9	Sweet Potatoes
5 Spinach	10	Lentils
Bad Foods: Fibroids		
Of the Foods Included in the Top 100		
Grass-Fed Beef		

compounds that may help regulate estrogen levels, potentially beneficial for individuals with fibroids, as these growths are influenced by estrogen. Salmon, rich in omega-3 fatty acids, possesses anti-inflammatory properties that may contribute to managing symptoms associated with fibroids by reducing inflammation and supporting overall reproductive health.

43. Hemorrhoids

Prevalence: 30.4 (per 1000 people in USA)

Hemorrhoids are painful, inflamed veins in the anus and lower rectum. Hemorrhoids have a long list of causes, however often times unknown. They are very common and can produce a great amount of discomfort. Pain, swelling, bleeding, itching, and irritation are common symptoms associated with hemorrhoids. Although not often serious, certain cases require medical attention to prevent serious complications such as anemia and blood clot

Top 10 Foods: Hemorrhoids			
All Wild Caught/Organic/Grass-Fed/etc			
1	Raspberries	6	Lentils
2	Apples	7	Brussel Sprouts
3	Whole Oats	8	Broccoli
4	Brown Rice	9	Strawberries
5	Black Beans	10	Blueberries

formation. Raspberries and apples, high in fiber, can aid in softening stools and promoting regular bowel movements, potentially reducing the risk of hemorrhoid development or exacerbation. Brown rice, also a good source of fiber, supports digestive health and may contribute to preventing constipation, a common factor associated with hemorrhoids.

44. Syncope

Prevalence: 28.9 (per 1000 people in USA)

Syncope is passing out or fainting often due to a sudden drop in heart rate and blood pressure. Types of syncope include vasovagal, situational, postural, neurologic, and sometimes unknown. Syncope can happen at any age and in both men and women. Syncope can often times be preceded by warning signs or can come without warning. Although manageable, it is important to be attentive to determining the underlying

Top 10 Foods: Syncope			
All Wild Caught/Organic/Grass-Fed/etc			
1	Spinach	6	Brown Rice
2	Bananas	7	Garlic Cloves
3	Salmon	8	Milk
4	Almonds	9	Grass-Fed Beef
5	Eggs	10	Cantaloupe

cause and managing it properly. Spinach and bananas, rich in potassium, contribute to maintaining proper electrolyte balance, potentially preventing syncope by supporting heart function and blood pressure regulation. Salmon, with its omega-3 fatty acids, may also aid in cardiovascular health, potentially reducing the risk of syncope episodes by promoting stable blood circulation and overall cardiovascular function.

45. Peripheral Arterial Disease

Prevalence: 25.8 (per 1000 people in USA)

Peripheral Arterial Disease (PAD) is a serious condition that leads to decreased circulation to limbs. This is often due to narrowing and blockage in arteries, reducing blood flow from providing oxygen and nutrients to the tissue in demand. This can lead to a varying range of symptoms such as mild pain and cold hands and feet to gangrene and limb loss. PAD needs to be taken seriously and requires immediate medical attention to prevent life

Top 10 Foods: Peripheral Artery Disease			
All Wild Caught/Organic/Grass-Fed/etc			
1	Broccoli	6	Spinach
2	Whole Oats	7	Apples
3	Walnuts	8	Kale
4	Barley	9	Almonds
5	Salmon	10	Oranges

threatening outcomes. Broccoli, whole oats, and walnuts are beneficial for individuals with peripheral arterial disease due to their content of fiber, antioxidants, and omega-3 fatty acids. These nutrients may help improve blood flow, reduce inflammation, and support overall cardiovascular health, potentially mitigating symptoms and complications associated with peripheral arterial disease.

46. Gout

Prevalence: 25.2 (per 1000 people in USA)

Gout is a common form of arthritis that can occur in various joints, most commonly the big toe joint. It typically presents as a red, hot, swollen joint with severe pain. Gout is caused by excess in uric acid levels which can be due to either overproduction or underexcretion. Gout can be managed by diet and medications however, it is important to determine the underlying cause to properly manage the condition. Almonds, whole oats, eggs, and oranges are suitable for individuals with gout as they offer a balance of protein, fiber, and vitamin C without significantly contributing to purine levels. These foods

Top 10 Foods: Gout			
All Wild Caught/Organic/Grass-Fed/etc			
1	Almonds	6	Avocados
2	Whole Oats	7	Cherries
3	Eggs	8	Salmon
4	Oranges	9	Mackerel
5	Walnuts	10	Chicken

Bad Foods: Gout	
Of the Foods Included in the Top 100	
Beef Liver	Sardines
Grass-Fed Beef	Tuna

may help manage gout symptoms by supporting a diet that minimizes purine intake while providing essential nutrients that contribute to overall health and may assist in preventing gout flare-ups.

47. Valvular Heart Disease

Prevalence: 25.0 (per 1000 people in USA)

Valvular heart disease is when one or more, out of four, valves of the heart do not function properly, disrupting the correct flow of blood through the heart. Severity of valvular heart disease can vary significantly and may require surgical repair or replacement. Signs and symptoms include abnormal heart sounds, chest pain, abdominal swelling, fatigue, shortness of breath, dizziness, and several others. There are various causes and types of

Top 10 Foods: Valvular Heart Disease			
All Wild Caught/Organic/Grass-Fed/etc			
1	Salmon	6	Walnuts
2	Mackerel	7	Herring
3	Almonds	8	Black Beans
4	Blueberries	9	Kale
5	Oranges	10	Broccoli

valvular heart disease and it is important to determine the condition and manage properly to prevent serious health issues. Salmon and mackerel, high in omega-3 fatty acids, may benefit individuals with valvular heart disease by supporting heart health and potentially reducing inflammation associated with the condition. Almonds, with their monounsaturated fats, and blueberries, rich in antioxidants, contribute to a heart-healthy diet, potentially promoting overall cardiovascular well-being and assisting in the management of valvular heart disease.

48. Psoriasis

Prevalence: 24.3 (per 1000 people in USA)

Psoriasis is a common skin condition that can cause scaling, red, itchy patches on extensor surfaces such as knees, elbows, trunk, and scalp. Psoriasis can also cause arthritic joints, pitting nails, sausage digits, and other skin changes. There are various types of psoriasis with a range of severity. If not managed properly, psoriasis can decrease quality of life and impact daily activities. Psoriasis is known to be caused by an immune system abnormality and can be triggered by several various factors. Proper medical management is very important in preventing serious complications. Salmon, abundant in omega-3

Top 10 Foods: Psoriasis			
All Wild Caught/Organic/Grass-Fed/etc			
1	Salmon	6	Blueberries
2	Spinach	7	Herring
3	Kale	8	Strawberries
4	Mackerel	9	Walnuts
5	Broccoli	10	Flaxseeds

Bad Foods: Psoriasis	
Of the Foods Included in the Top 100	
Bell Peppers	Eggplant
Eggs	Potatoes

fatty acids, and spinach and broccoli, rich in vitamins A and C, possess anti-inflammatory properties that may be beneficial for individuals with psoriasis by helping manage inflammation and supporting skin health. Additionally, these foods contribute to a nutrient-dense diet that may positively impact overall well-being and potentially alleviate symptoms associated with psoriasis.

49. Aortic Aneurysm

Prevalence: 22.0 (per 1000 people in USA)

An aortic aneurysm is an abnormal bulge that occurs in the wall of the aorta, which is a major blood vessel that carries blood from the heart to the rest of the body. This can occur anywhere along the aorta and can come in tube form or round. The types of aortic aneurysm include abdominal or thoracic based on their anatomical location. Aortic aneurysms can lead to very serious complications such as tears, weakening of the

Top 10 Foods: Aortic Aneurysm			
All Wild Caught/Organic/Grass-Fed/etc			
1	Apples	6	Grapefruit
2	Bananas	7	Limes
3	Oranges	8	Salmon
4	Pears	9	Almonds
5	Lemons	10	Brown Rice

walls of the aorta, or ruptures. Proper medical management is very important in preventing dangerous complications. Apples, bananas, and oranges, rich in fiber and antioxidants, contribute to cardiovascular health by promoting stable blood pressure and reducing oxidative stress, which may be beneficial for individuals with aortic aneurysms. Including these fruits in the diet supports overall heart health and may contribute to the prevention of complications associated with aortic aneurysms.

50. Heart Failure

Prevalence: 19.8 (per 1000 people in USA)

Heart failure, often referred to as congestive heart failure, is when the heart muscle fails to function properly and pump blood efficiently. Signs and symptoms include weakness, fatigue, loss of appetite, nausea, swelling, irregular heartbeat, chest pain, shortness of breath, and many other symptoms. Heart failure is a serious condition and can be life threatening. Although not all conditions leading to heart failure can be cured, lifestyle

Top 10 Foods: Heart Failure			
All Wild Caught/Organic/Grass-Fed/etc			
1	Salmon	6	Walnuts
2	Mackerel	7	Herring
3	Almonds	8	Black Beans
4	Blueberries	9	Kale
5	Oranges	10	Broccoli

changes can significantly help improve quality of life and heart function. Salmon, rich in omega-3 fatty acids, almonds containing monounsaturated fats, and oranges with their vitamin C content contribute to heart health by supporting proper circulation, reducing inflammation, and maintaining blood vessel integrity, potentially benefiting individuals with heart failure. Additionally, black beans, high in fiber and potassium, can be part of a heart-healthy diet, assisting in managing fluid balance and blood pressure for those with heart failure.

51. Conjunctivitis

Prevalence: 18.2 (per 1000 people in USA)

Conjunctivitis (pink eye) is an inflammation or infection of the transparent membrane (conjunctiva) that lines the eyelid and covers the white part of the eye. Conjunctivitis can occur at any age and in both men and women. It is normally caused by a viral or bacterial infection, or an allergic reaction. In babies it commonly occurs due an incompletely open tear duct. Signs and symptoms include redness, itching, burning, discharge, and tearing. Conjunctivitis can often create serious discomfort. Spinach and carrots, rich in vitamins A and C, along with grapefruit containing antioxidants, contribute to eye health and may be beneficial for individuals with conjunctivitis by supporting the immune system and reducing inflammation. These nutrient-dense foods provide essential nutrients that play a role in maintaining overall eye function and potentially alleviating symptoms associated with conjunctivitis.

Top 10 Foods: Conjunctivitis			
All Wild Caught/Organic/Grass-Fed/etc			
1	Spinach	6	Eggs
2	Kale	7	Oranges
3	Carrots	8	Sweet Potatoes
4	Grapefruit	9	Tomatoes
5	Broccoli	10	Strawberries

Bad Foods: Conjunctivitis	
Of the Foods Included in the Top 100	
Potatoes	

52. ADHD

Prevalence: 18.2 (per 1000 people in USA)

Attention deficit hyperactivity disorder (ADHD) is a mental health disorder that can cause excessive hyperactive and impulsive behaviors. People with ADHD often have trouble focusing their attention on a single task or being still for extended periods of time. ADHD can routinely affect daily performance, productivity, and quality of life. Management of ADHD is important in maintaining a normal lifestyle. Attention Deficit Disorder (ADD) is a type of ADHD that does not involve hyperactivity. Salmon, rich in omega-3 fatty acids, along with spinach and eggs containing essential nutrients like iron and B vitamins, may support cognitive function and attention in individuals with ADHD. Flaxseeds, a source of omega-3s and fiber, can also contribute to a balanced diet that supports brain health, potentially providing benefits for those managing ADHD symptoms.

Top 10 Foods: ADHD			
All Wild Caught/Organic/Grass-Fed/etc			
1	Salmon	6	Herring
2	Spinach	7	Black Beans
3	Eggs	8	Flaxseeds
4	Mackerel	9	Kidney Beans
5	Chicken	10	Chickpeas

53. Menopause

Prevalence: 17.7 (per 1000 people in USA)

Menopause occurs when women have stopped menstruating for about 12 months after a certain age, on average about 51 years old in the United States. Although a natural course of life in women, physical and emotional symptoms can hinder quality of life, performance, and impact daily activity. Signs and symptoms of menopause include irregular periods, hot flashes, vaginal dryness, mood changes, chills, night sweats, and many others. Symptoms often vary from individual to individual but certain dietary changes can help maintain quality of life. Proper foods contribute to hormonal balance, provide essential nutrients, and possess anti-inflammatory properties, potentially supporting overall well-being during the menopausal transition.

Top 10 Foods: Menopause			
All Wild Caught/Organic/Grass-Fed/etc			
1	Salmon	6	Sardines
2	Broccoli	7	Flaxseeds
3	Mackerel	8	Chia Seeds
4	Almonds	9	Chickpeas
5	Eggs	10	Blueberries

Bad Foods: Menopause	
Of the Foods Included in the Top 100	
Red Wine	

54. Alzheimer's / Dementia

Prevalence: 17.6 (per 1000 people in USA)

Alzheimer's is the most common cause of dementia. Genetics certainly plays a role in how our brain functions, develops, and in the case of Alzheimer's, deteriorates. However, several lifestyle and nutritional changes can prevent the development or slow down the progression of Alzheimer's. Alzheimer's is known to significantly lower quality of life, decrease functionality, and impact day to day activity. It is important to manage the physical and mental effects of Alzheimer's properly. Spinach and strawberries, rich in antioxidants and vitamins, along with salmon containing omega-3 fatty acids, may support brain health and potentially reduce the risk of Alzheimer's disease. These foods contribute to a nutrient-dense diet that promotes cognitive function, provides essential nutrients, and has anti-inflammatory properties, which are factors associated with maintaining brain health and reducing the risk of neurodegenerative disorders like Alzheimer's.

Top 10 Foods: Alzheimer's / Dementia			
All Wild Caught/Organic/Grass-Fed/etc			
1	Spinach	6	Blueberries
2	Strawberries	7	Herring
3	Salmon	8	Dark Chocolate
4	Kale	9	Almonds
5	Mackerel	10	Oranges

Bad Foods: Alzheimer's / Dementia	
Of the Foods Included in the Top 100	
Grass-Fed Beef	

55. Bipolar Disorder

Prevalence: 17.3 (per 1000 people in USA)

Bipolar disorder is a mental health condition that exhibits extreme mood swings of mania and depression. The manic phase of bipolar often resembles as euphoria, high energy, agitated, and irritable while the depressive phase presents with sadness, lack of interest, and hopelessness. A great deal of variability exists in frequency, intensity, and episodes of mood swings. Bipolar disorder can have a significant impact on quality of life,

Top 10 Foods: Bipolar Disorder			
All Wild Caught/Organic/Grass-Fed/etc			
1	Salmon	6	Chickpeas
2	Mackerel	7	Cheese
3	Whole Oats	8	Dark Chocolate
4	Herring	9	Quinoa
5	Lentils	10	Spinach

performance, relationships, and impede daily activities. Proper management can help improve quality of life. Salmon and mackerel, rich in omega-3 fatty acids, along with whole oats and lentils containing complex carbohydrates and essential nutrients, may be beneficial for individuals with bipolar disorder. These foods contribute to a balanced diet that supports brain function, provides steady energy levels, and potentially helps manage mood swings associated with bipolar disorder by promoting stable blood sugar and neurotransmitter levels.

56. Iron Deficiency Anemia

Prevalence: 15.2 (per 1000 people in USA)

Anemia is a common condition in which the blood lacks enough healthy red blood cells or hemoglobin, in this case due to low iron. Red blood cells carry oxygen to all our organs and tissues with the help of hemoglobin and iron. Anemia can lead to several symptoms due to lack oxygen delivery to our organs and tissues. Iron, vitamin B12, folate, vitamin C, and other nutritional factors can help reduce symptoms of anemia. Variety of symptoms

Top 10 Foods: Iron Deficiency Anemia			
All Wild Caught/Organic/Grass-Fed/etc			
1	Spinach	6	Kale
2	Tomatoes	7	Broccoli
3	Grass-Fed Beef	8	Black Beans
4	Soybeans	9	Kidney Beans
5	Beef Liver	10	Chickpeas

can occur due to iron deficiency anemia, but with proper management, quality of life can be maintained. Spinach and tomatoes, rich in vitamin C, enhance the absorption of non-heme iron found in plant-based sources, which can be beneficial for individuals with iron deficiency anemia. Beef and beef liver, excellent sources of heme iron, contribute to increasing iron levels more efficiently, aiding in the management of anemia by supplying readily absorbable iron to the body.

57. Peptic Ulcer

Prevalence: 13.7 (per 1000 people in USA)

Peptic ulcers (stomach ulcers) are open sores that develop on the inside lining of the stomach and the upper portion of the small intestine resulting in stomach pain, bloating, food intolerance, heartburn, nausea, and other symptoms. Causes include certain medications, H. Pylori bacteria, alcohol, stress, spicy food, and many others. Although manageable, peptic ulcers can have serious complications such as perforation, internal bleeding, obstruction, and gastric cancer. Peptic ulcers should be managed properly and given attention if encountered. Salmon, with its omega-3 fatty acids, blueberries

Top 10 Foods: Peptic Ulcer			
All Wild Caught/Organic/Grass-Fed/etc			
1	Salmon	6	Bell Peppers
2	Broccoli	7	Cabbage
3	Blueberries	8	Turmeric Root
4	Whole Oats	9	Grapes
5	Greek Yogurt	10	

Bad Foods: Peptic Ulcer	
Of the Foods Included in the Top 100	
Chili Peppers	Red Wine
Dark Chocolate	Tomatoes
Grass-Fed Beef	

containing antioxidants, and Greek yogurt providing probiotics, can contribute to a diet that may support the healing of peptic ulcers. These foods possess anti-inflammatory and gut-friendly properties, potentially aiding in the reduction of inflammation and promoting a balanced gut microbiome, which is crucial for managing and preventing peptic ulcer symptoms.

58. Contact Dermatitis

Prevalence: 13.6 (per 1000 people in USA)

Contact dermatitis is a skin condition that presents with a red, itchy rash caused by direct contact with a substance or an allergic reaction to a certain allergen. Symptoms include burning, swelling, redness, itchiness, scaling, blister formation, and tenderness. These symptoms can appear as soon minutes to hours after exposure to the irritant. Although normally contact dermatitis does not often produce serious complications, it can cause

Top 10 Foods: Contact Dermatitis			
All Wild Caught/Organic/Grass-Fed/etc			
1	Salmon	6	Broccoli
2	Mackerel	7	Walnuts
3	Herring	8	Flaxseeds
4	Spinach	9	Cherries
5	Kale	10	Kefir

significant discomfort. Salmon, mackerel, and herring, rich in omega-3 fatty acids, along with spinach containing vitamins and antioxidants, and walnuts with anti-inflammatory properties, may collectively contribute to reducing inflammation and supporting skin health in individuals with contact dermatitis. These foods can be beneficial in managing the immune response and promoting overall skin well-being, potentially alleviating symptoms associated with contact dermatitis.

59. Chronic Liver Disease / Cirrhosis

Prevalence: 13.4 (per 1000 people in USA)

Chronic liver disease is a progressive process in which recurrent destruction and regeneration of the organ leads to eventual fibrosis and cirrhosis. Liver, being one of the most important organs in the body, has many roles. Chronic liver disease can have very serious symptoms and complications that can eventually lead to hepatocellular carcinoma, liver failure, and even death. Maintaining a healthy liver is crucial to healthy living and preventing serious complications and preserving a good quality of life. Broccoli, almonds, and garlic are rich in antioxidants

Top 10 Foods: Chronic Liver Disease			
All Wild Caught/Organic/Grass-Fed/etc			
1	Broccoli	6	Extra Virgin Olive Oil
2	Almonds	7	Grapefruit
3	Garlic Cloves	8	Beets
4	Lemons	9	Salmon
5	Avocados	10	Blueberries
Bad Foods: Chronic Liver Disease			
Of the Foods Included in the Top 100			
Red Wine			

and anti-inflammatory compounds, potentially supporting liver health and mitigating inflammation associated with cirrhosis. Avocados, along with extra virgin olive oil, provide healthy fats and may aid in managing cirrhosis by promoting a balanced diet that supports liver function and overall well-being.

60. Inguinal Hernia

Prevalence: 12.8 (per 1000 people in USA)

An Inguinal hernia is when part of the intestine protrudes (herniates) through the abdominal wall near the groin area. An inguinal hernia can be very painful. Normally it is noticed the most when one exerts themselves coughing, lifting heavy objects, or bending over. Although often times not dangerous, inguinal hernias can have serious complications. They can certainly decrease quality of life, performance, and impede day

Top 10 Foods: Inguinal Hernia			
All Wild Caught/Organic/Grass-Fed/etc			
1	Peas	6	Pears
2	Whole Oats	7	Spinach
3	Ginger Root	8	Apples
4	Brown Rice	9	Kale
5	Quinoa	10	Collard Greens

to day activities. Therefore, it is a condition that needs to be properly managed. Peas, whole oats, and ginger root are beneficial for individuals with inguinal hernia due to their high fiber content, potentially aiding in regular bowel movements and preventing constipation, which can exacerbate hernia symptoms. Additionally, ginger root, known for its anti-inflammatory properties, may help alleviate inflammation and discomfort associated with inguinal hernias.

61. Constipation

Prevalence: 12.1 (per 1000 people in USA)

Constipation is difficult passage of stool or infrequent bowel movements, oftentimes defined as less than three bowel movements per week. Constipation is normally diagnosed when it lasts a few weeks or longer.

Constipation is widely experienced amongst individuals, however, when it becomes a chronic or frequent problem, constipation can hinder an individual's daily activity and significantly lower quality of life. Several

Top 10 Foods: Constipation			
All Wild Caught/Organic/Grass-Fed/etc			
1	Flaxseeds	6	Broccoli
2	Pears	7	Whole Oats
3	Prunes	8	Greek Yogurt
4	Spinach	9	Raspberries
5	Apples	10	Chia Seeds

nutritional and dietary changes can help reduce constipation and increase quality of life. Flaxseeds, pears, and prunes are excellent natural remedies for constipation as they are rich in fiber, promoting regular bowel movements and preventing digestive discomfort. These foods can contribute to improved digestion by adding bulk to the stool and aiding in the softening and passage of stool, supporting overall digestive health and relieving constipation.

62. Hyperthyroidism

Prevalence: 12.0 (per 1000 people in USA)

Hyperthyroidism is a medical condition where the thyroid produces thyroxine, leading to increased metabolism, weight loss, and irregular or rapid heart rhythm. Other signs and symptoms include anxiety, increased appetite, palpitations, nervousness, tremors, sweating, heat intolerance, changes in menstrual pattern, difficulty sleeping, and many others. It is important to manage hyperthyroidism properly in order to

Top 10 Foods: Hyperthyroidism			
All Wild Caught/Organic/Grass-Fed/etc			
1	Eggs	6	Spinach
2	Seaweed	7	Kale
3	Brazil Nuts	8	Chicken
4	Greek Yogurt	9	Sardines
5	Salmon	10	Milk

maintain quality of life, performance, happiness, and daily activity. Eggs, seaweed, and Brazil nuts are beneficial for individuals with hyperthyroidism as they provide essential nutrients like selenium and iodine, supporting thyroid function. Selenium, found in Brazil nuts, and iodine, present in seaweed, play crucial roles in thyroid hormone production and regulation, while eggs contribute protein and essential amino acids that support overall thyroid health.

63. Schizophrenia

Prevalence: 12.0 (per 1000 people in USA)

Schizophrenia is a debilitating mental condition that often results in combination of hallucinations, delusions, and extremely disordered thinking and behavior that impairs daily function. There is no true cure for Schizophrenia, but proper lifelong management can help improve hallucinations, thoughts, delusions, and ultimately, performance, mental and physical health, relationships, daily function, and

Top 10 Foods: Schizophrenia			
All Wild Caught/Organic/Grass-Fed/etc			
1	Salmon	6	Apples
2	Mackerel	7	Kale
3	Herring	8	Broccoli
4	Spinach	9	Chicken
5	Asparagus	10	Almonds

quality of life. People with Schizophrenia require professional, personal, supportive, and dietary help to be able to manage their day-to-day activities. Salmon, mackerel, and herring, rich in omega-3 fatty acids, along with spinach containing folate and apples providing antioxidants, may contribute to a nutrient-dense diet that supports brain health and may have potential benefits for individuals with schizophrenia. These foods provide essential nutrients that play a role in neurotransmitter function, anti-inflammatory effects, and overall mental well-being, potentially aiding in the management of symptoms associated with schizophrenia.

64. Pregnancy

Prevalence: 11.1 (per 1000 people in USA)

Although pregnancy and childbirth are a natural part of life, many adverse symptoms are associated throughout pregnancy. The list of mental and physical signs and symptoms of pregnancy is endless. In addition, keeping a healthy lifestyle and diet is vital for the health of both the mother and the baby. Specific foods can help maintain a healthy lifestyle and quality of life, and prevent adverse outcomes and long list of complications associated with pregnancy. Kale, rich in folate and iron, along with eggs providing protein and essential nutrients, and lentils offering

Top 10 Foods: Pregnancy			
All Wild Caught/Organic/Grass-Fed/etc			
1	Kale	6	Broccoli
2	Eggs	7	Whole Oats
3	Lentils	8	Chicken
4	Salmon	9	Greek Yogurt
5	Spinach	10	Sweet Potatoes
Bad Foods: Pregnancy			
Of the Foods Included in the Top 100			
Red Wine			

folate and iron, form a nutritious combination beneficial for pregnancy. These foods contribute to the development of the fetal nervous system, support the increased blood volume during pregnancy, and provide essential nutrients that are crucial for the health and well-being of both the mother and the developing baby.

65. Epilepsy

Prevalence: 10.8 (per 1000 people in USA)

Epilepsy is a serious neurological (central nervous system) disorder in which brain activity becomes irregular, causing seizures or periods of unusual behavior, sensations, and sometimes loss of awareness. People with epilepsy can show a range of signs and symptoms. Epilepsy affects both male and female of all ages. It can present itself differently and with various severity. Epilepsy can certainly decrease quality of life,

Top 10 Foods: Epilepsy			
All Wild Caught/Organic/Grass-Fed/etc			
1	Broccoli	6	Spinach
2	Strawberries	7	Kale
3	Eggs	8	Mackerel
4	Blueberries	9	Almonds
5	Raspberries	10	Avocados

performance, and impede day to day activities. Epilepsy can cause serious complications and proper management is essential.

Broccoli, strawberries, eggs, and raspberries are valuable for individuals with epilepsy as they contain important nutrients such as vitamin B6, antioxidants, and omega-3 fatty acids that support brain health. Including these foods in the diet may contribute to maintaining stable brain function and reducing the risk or severity of seizures associated with epilepsy.

66. Cancer: Breast

Prevalence: 10.8 (per 1000 people in USA)

Breast cancer is one of the most common cancers encountered in the United States. Signs and symptoms include breast mass or lump, abnormal changes in appearance, pigmentation, scaling, abnormal discharge, and many more. Various factors have been associated with development of abnormal growth of cells in the breast, leading to breast cancer. These cells can divide, grow rapidly, and metastasize to other parts of the body. Breast cancer can significantly affect quality of life. Proper management of breast cancer is crucial to prevent severe outcomes

Top 10 Foods: Cancer: Breast			
All Wild Caught/Organic/Grass-Fed/etc			
1	Kale	6	Broccoli
2	Carrots	7	Strawberries
3	Green Tea	8	Whole Oats
4	Salmon	9	Blueberries
5	Mackerel	10	Brown Rice

Bad Foods: Cancer: Breast	
Of the Foods Included in the Top 100	
Grass-Fed Beef	Red Wine

and complications. Kale and carrots, rich in antioxidants and phytochemicals, along with salmon providing omega-3 fatty acids and green tea containing polyphenols, collectively contribute to a diet that may be protective against breast cancer. These foods possess anti-inflammatory properties, support immune function, and may help regulate hormone levels, potentially reducing the risk of breast cancer and promoting overall breast health.

67. Hepatitis C

Prevalence: 10.2 (per 1000 people in USA)

Hepatitis C is a viral infection caused by hepatitis C virus (HCV) that is transmitted through infected blood. Hepatitis C mainly affects the liver, leading to damage and inflammation, and ultimately serious complications. Signs and symptoms include bleeding or bruising easily, jaundice, fatigue, swelling, weight loss, ascites, dark urine, and many others. If left untreated, Hepatitis C can become a chronic condition resulting in liver cirrhosis, hepatocellular carcinoma, and liver failure. Hepatitis C infection is a very serious and common condition and proper management

Top 10 Foods: Hepatitis C			
All Wild Caught/Organic/Grass-Fed/etc			
1	Kale	6	Almonds
2	Salmon	7	Whole Oats
3	Spinach	8	Walnuts
4	Mackerel	9	Garlic Cloves
5	Broccoli	10	Herring
Bad Foods: Hepatitis C			
Of the Foods Included in the Top 100			
Grass-Fed Beef			

is critical. Kale, salmon, and spinach are beneficial for individuals with hepatitis C as they offer essential nutrients like vitamins, antioxidants, and omega-3 fatty acids, which may support liver health and immune function. These foods, when included in a well-balanced diet, can contribute to the management of hepatitis C by providing key nutrients that aid in reducing inflammation and promoting overall liver function.

68. Cancer: Prostate

Prevalence: 9.6 (per 1000 people in USA)

Prostate cancer is a very common cancer among men in the United State. Signs and symptoms include painful and abnormal urination, blood in urine or semen, discomfort, and many more. Various factors have been associated with development of abnormal growth of cells in the prostate, leading to prostate cancer. These cells can divide, grow rapidly, and metastasize to other parts of the body. Prostate cancer can significantly affect quality of life. Proper management of prostate cancer is crucial to prevent severe outcomes and complications. Tomatoes, rich

Top 10 Foods: Cancer: Prostate			
All Wild Caught/Organic/Grass-Fed/etc			
1	Tomatoes	6	Cauliflower
2	Salmon	7	Almonds
3	Mackerel	8	Brussel Sprouts
4	Broccoli	9	Strawberries
5	Herring	10	Blueberries
Bad Foods: Cancer: Prostate			
Of the Foods Included in the Top 100			
Grass-Fed Beef			

in lycopene, and fatty fish such as salmon and mackerel, high in omega-3 fatty acids, along with brussels sprouts containing sulforaphane, contribute to a prostate-healthy diet. These foods have shown potential in reducing the risk of prostate cancer due to their anti-inflammatory and antioxidant properties, supporting overall prostate health and potentially aiding in cancer prevention.

69. Inflammatory Bowel Disease

Prevalence: 9.3 (per 1000 people in USA)

Inflammatory bowel disease (IBD), which includes Crohn's and Ulcerative Colitis, is a chronic inflammatory condition of the digestive tract, resulting in many unpleasant symptoms and a decline in quality of life. Some of these signs and symptoms include diarrhea, abdominal pain, cramping, bloating, fever, fatigue, weight loss, and many more. A good diet can help maintain a healthy lifestyle and quality of life, and prevent

Top 10 Foods: Inflammatory Bowel Disease			
All Wild Caught/Organic/Grass-Fed/etc			
1	Soybeans	6	Eggs
2	Salmon	7	Greek Yogurt
3	Mackerel	8	Herring
4	Broccoli	9	Black Beans
5	Whole Oats	10	Chickpeas

adverse outcomes and long list of symptoms and serious complications associated with Inflammatory Bowel Disease. Soybeans, salmon, broccoli, and whole oats are beneficial for individuals with inflammatory bowel disease (IBD) as they provide a combination of omega-3 fatty acids, fiber, and antioxidants that may help reduce inflammation and support gut health. These foods can contribute to a well-rounded diet that aids in managing symptoms of IBD by promoting a balanced inflammatory response and maintaining digestive wellness.

70. Obsessive Compulsive Disorder

Prevalence: 9.2 (per 1000 people in USA)

OCD involves repeated thoughts, fears, obsessions, and behaviors that if not executed by an individual with OCD, it results in great distress and anxiety. Oftentimes, despite executing these obsessive compulsions, individuals with OCD tend to continue to feel anxious and distressed. This can result in creating cycles or rituals for individuals with OCD. Severity of OCD varies amongst individuals and is a prevalent problem in the

Top 10 Foods: OCD			
All Wild Caught/Organic/Grass-Fed/etc			
1	Almonds	6	Salmon
2	Spinach	7	Mackerel
3	Swiss Chard	8	Chicken
4	Grass-Fed Beef	9	Whole Oats
5	Seaweed	10	Blueberries

United States. OCD can greatly impact an individual's daily activity and quality of life. Several nutritional and dietary changes can help reduce the symptoms of OCD. Almonds, swiss chard, and beef contain nutrients such as magnesium, iron, and zinc, which play roles in neurotransmitter regulation and may contribute to managing symptoms of obsessive-compulsive disorder (OCD). Including these foods in a balanced diet may support overall mental health by providing essential minerals that can positively influence brain function and potentially alleviate symptoms associated with OCD.

71. Anemia of Chronic Disease

Prevalence: 9.1 (per 1000 people in USA)

Anemia of Chronic Disease is a common condition in which the blood lacks enough healthy red blood cells or hemoglobin. Red blood cells carry oxygen to all our organs and tissues with the help of hemoglobin. Anemia can lead to several symptoms due to lack oxygen delivery to our organs and tissues. Iron, vitamin B12, folate, vitamin C, and other nutritional factors can help reduce symptoms of anemia. Variety of symptoms can occur due to anemia of chronic disease, but with proper management, quality of life can be maintained. Spinach, kidney beans, and beef

Top 10 Foods: Anemia of Chronic Disease			
All Wild Caught/Organic/Grass-Fed/etc			
1	Spinach	6	Beef Liver
2	Kidney Beans	7	Kale
3	Chick Peas	8	Chicken
4	Grass-Fed Beef	9	Tomatoes
5	Oysters	10	Sardines

Bad Foods: Anemia of Chronic Disease	
Of the Foods Included in the Top 100	
Barley	Green Tea
Brown Rice	Whole Oats

are excellent choices for individuals with anemia of chronic disease as they contain iron, a crucial component for red blood cell production, and vitamin B12, which supports the synthesis of hemoglobin. These foods contribute to addressing nutritional deficiencies often associated with chronic diseases, promoting optimal blood cell function and aiding in the management of anemia.

72. Pneumonia

Prevalence: 9.1 (per 1000 people in USA)

Pneumonia is an infection (bacterial, fungal, viral) that results in inflammation of air sacs in the lungs, causing them to often be filled with fluid or pus. People with pneumonia experience shortness of breath, fever, chills, cough with phlegm, and significant discomfort when breathing. Severity varies a great amount in pneumonia but in infants, older individuals, and people with a compromised immune system, it can be life threatening. Proper management is critical in avoiding serious complications. Pneumonia can significantly impact one's quality of life

Top 10 Foods: Pneumonia			
All Wild Caught/Organic/Grass-Fed/etc			
1	Ginger Root	6	Mackerel
2	Salmon	7	Strawberries
3	Garlic Cloves	8	Blueberries
4	Turmeric Root	9	Avocados
5	Kale	10	Herring

Bad Foods: Pneumonia	
Of the Foods Included in the Top 100	
Milk	

and performance. Ginger root, salmon, garlic, and turmeric root are beneficial for pneumonia due to their anti-inflammatory and immune-boosting properties. These foods may aid in reducing inflammation, supporting respiratory health, and strengthening the immune system, potentially assisting in the recovery process from pneumonia.

73. Glaucoma

Prevalence: 8.2 (per 1000 people in USA)

Glaucoma is an eye condition that results in damage to the optic nerve, often due to an abnormally high pressure in the eyes. Glaucoma tends to occur over time and gradually, showing minimal to no signs until reaching late stages of the disease. Because of this, getting routine eye exams, using eye protection, and taking preventative measures is important. Glaucoma can occur at any age but is more common in older adults. It is one

Top 10 Foods: Glaucoma			
All Wild Caught/Organic/Grass-Fed/etc			
1	Oranges	6	Carrots
2	Kale	7	Lemons
3	Dark Chocolate	8	Herring
4	Salmon	9	Sweet Potatoes
5	Mackerel	10	Grapefruit

of the leading causes of blindness in people over the age of 60. Glaucoma can significantly impact one's quality of life and performance. Oranges, kale, dark chocolate, and salmon are beneficial for individuals with glaucoma as they contain nutrients such as vitamin C, antioxidants, and omega-3 fatty acids that may support eye health and help manage intraocular pressure. Including these foods in the diet can contribute to a well-rounded approach to supporting overall eye function and potentially mitigating the progression of glaucoma.

74. Fibromyalgia

Prevalence: 8.2 (per 1000 people in USA)

Fibromyalgia is a condition characterized by widespread musculoskeletal pain along with fatigue, sleep, memory, and mood issues. It is believed that fibromyalgia magnifies painful sensations by affecting the way the brain and spinal cord process painful and nonpainful stimuli. Symptoms often begin after physical trauma, surgery, infection or significant psychological stress. Symptoms can also gradually accrue over time with no single

Top 10 Foods: Fibromyalgia			
All Wild Caught/Organic/Grass-Fed/etc			
1	Salmon	6	Mackerel
2	Spinach	7	Almonds
3	Kale	8	Brown Rice
4	Collard Greens	9	Walnuts
5	Tuna	10	Greek Yogurt

triggering event. Fibromyalgia can significantly impact one's quality of life and performance. Salmon, spinach, and tuna are beneficial for individuals with fibromyalgia due to their rich content of omega-3 fatty acids, antioxidants, and anti-inflammatory properties. These foods may contribute to managing symptoms associated with fibromyalgia by potentially reducing inflammation and supporting overall joint and muscle health.

75. Pelvic Inflammatory Disease

Prevalence: 7.9 (per 1000 people in USA)

Pelvic Inflammatory Disease (PID) is an infection that results in inflammation of the female reproductive organs. It most often follows when sexually transmitted bacteria spread to the uterus, fallopian tubes or ovaries. Severity of symptoms can vary significantly. Signs and symptoms include pain, abnormal bleeding, abnormal discharge, abnormal urination, fever, chills, and many others. Proper management of PID is important to prevent severe outcomes and complications. PID can decrease quality of life, performance, and impede day to day activities. Salmon is

Top 10 Foods: Pelvic Inflammatory Disease			
All Wild Caught/Organic/Grass-Fed/etc			
1	Salmon	6	Extra Virgin Olive Oil
2	Spinach	7	Flaxseeds
3	Almonds	8	Walnuts
4	Blueberries	9	Sardines
5	Herring	10	Turmeric Root

Bad Foods: Pelvic Inflammatory Disease	
Of the Foods Included in the Top 100	
Cheese	Milk
Grass-Fed Beef	Whole Wheat

beneficial for individuals with pelvic inflammatory disease due to its rich content of omega-3 fatty acids, which possess anti-inflammatory properties that may help manage symptoms associated with the condition. Almonds are beneficial for individuals with pelvic inflammatory disease as they provide essential nutrients like vitamin E and anti-inflammatory compounds that may support immune function

76. Congenital Heart Defect

Prevalence: 7.7 (per 1000 people in USA)

Congenital Heart Defect is a common birth defect where there is one or multiple flaws in the structure of the heart at birth. Severity can vary from having no long-term issues to having life-threatening complications. Signs and symptoms of congenital heart defects can present early or during adulthood. These abnormal heart rhythms (arrhythmias), cyanosis, shortness of breath, fatigue, generalized swelling, and many others. It can

Top 10 Foods: Congenital Heart Defect			
All Wild Caught/Organic/Grass-Fed/etc			
1	Salmon	6	Walnuts
2	Mackerel	7	Herring
3	Almonds	8	Black Beans
4	Blueberries	9	Kale
5	Oranges	10	Broccoli

decrease quality of life, performance, and impede day to day activities. Proper management is important to prevent severe complications.

Salmon, rich in omega-3 fatty acids, along with blueberries and oranges containing antioxidants and vitamin C, contribute to a heart-healthy diet that may benefit individuals with congenital heart defects. These foods support cardiovascular health, potentially aiding in managing inflammation and oxidative stress associated with congenital heart defects and promoting overall heart well-being.

77. Celiac Disease

Prevalence: 7.5 (per 1000 people in USA)

Celiac disease is a common condition where there is an immune response in the small intestine to gluten, a protein found in wheat, barley, and rye. Repeated exposure to gluten when having Celiac disease can damage the lining of the small intestine and prevents it from functioning properly and malabsorption. Symptoms include diarrhea, anemia, weight loss, mouth ulcers fatigue, abdominal pain, joint pain, osteoporosis, bloating and gas, constipation, nausea, vomiting, and many others. Celiac disease can decrease quality of life, performance, and impede day to day activities. Chickpeas, quinoa, and buckwheat are excellent choices for individuals with celiac disease as they are naturally gluten-free, providing essential nutrients and fiber without triggering gluten-related symptoms.

Top 10 Foods: Celiac Disease			
All Wild Caught/Organic/Grass-Fed/etc			
1	Chickpeas	6	Chicken
2	Quinoa	7	Almonds
3	Buckwheat	8	Eggs
4	Amaranth	9	Walnuts
5	Broccoli	10	Avocados

Bad Foods: Celiac Disease	
Of the Foods Included in the Top 100	
Barley	Whole Wheat

78. Hypothyroidism

Prevalence: 6.7 (per 1000 people in USA)

Hypothyroidism is a condition in which the thyroid gland does not produce enough thyroid hormone. Symptoms can include weight gain, depression, fatigue, dry skin, thinning hair, impaired memory, and others. To help prevent or slow down the progression of hypothyroidism, several nutrients can certainly play a significant role. For instance, iodine is an essential mineral required to produce thyroid hormones. Selenium, zinc, and some other vitamins can also play a role. It is also important to learn to avoid certain foods when it comes to hypothyroidism. Seaweed and Brazil nuts are beneficial for hypothyroidism as they are rich sources of iodine and selenium, respectively, essential minerals that support thyroid function. Including these foods in the diet may contribute to maintaining optimal thyroid health by providing the necessary nutrients for hormone production and regulation.

Top 10 Foods: Hypothyroidism			
All Wild Caught/Organic/Grass-Fed/etc			
1	Seaweed	6	Sardines
2	Brazil Nuts	7	Milk
3	Greek Yogurt	8	Grass-Fed Beef
4	Chicken	9	Tuna
5	Eggs	10	Oysters

Bad Foods: Hypothyroidism	
Of the Foods Included in the Top 100	
Brussel Sprouts	Cauliflower
Cabbage	Soybeans

79. Gastritis

Prevalence: 5.9 (per 1000 people in USA)

Gastritis is the inflammation of the lining of the stomach. Gastritis can be caused by infection, overuse of NSAIDs, and alcohol overuse. Gastritis can be acute or chronic. Symptoms include nausea, vomiting, abdominal pain, bloating, and indigestion. However, Gastritis can be asymptomatic at times. Gastritis affects many individuals in the United States annually. Although not often consequential, it can result in serious complications if not treated. A proper diet is essential in managing Gastritis. Greek yogurt, apples, and lentils are suitable for individuals with gastritis as they provide a combination of probiotics, fiber, and easily digestible proteins. These foods may contribute to a soothing and nourishing diet, potentially alleviating symptoms of gastritis by promoting a balanced gut environment and supporting overall digestive health.

Top 10 Foods: Gastritis			
All Wild Caught/Organic/Grass-Fed/etc			
1	Greek Yogurt	6	Blueberries
2	Lentils	7	Black Beans
3	Apples	8	Turmeric Root
4	Strawberries	9	Salmon
5	Ginger Root	10	Spinach

Bad Foods: Gastritis	
Of the Foods Included in the Top 100	
Chili Peppers	Limes
Dark Chocolate	Red Wine
Grapefruit	Tomatoes
Lemons	

80. Type I Diabetes

Prevalence: 5.5 (per 1000 people in USA)

Type 1 diabetes is a chronic condition in which the pancreas produces little or no insulin. Insulin is a hormone needed to absorb glucose to enter cells to produce energy. Even though most times it starts during childhood or adolescence, it can develop in adulthood. Symptoms include frequent urination, increased thirst, extreme hunger, irritability and other mood changes, weight loss, fatigue, and many others. Type 1 diabetes can decrease quality of life, performance, and impede day to day activities. Proper management is important to prevent severe outcomes. Strawberries and Greek yogurt are beneficial for individuals with type 1 diabetes as they offer a low-glycemic index and a combination of fiber, antioxidants, and protein, helping regulate blood sugar levels. Incorporating these foods into the diet may contribute to stable glucose levels and overall glycemic control in individuals managing type 1 diabetes.

Top 10 Foods: Type I Diabetes			
All Wild Caught/Organic/Grass-Fed/etc			
1	Strawberries	6	Mackerel
2	Greek Yogurt	7	Blueberries
3	Salmon	8	Herring
4	Spinach	9	Extra Virgin Olive Oil
5	Kale	10	Tomatoes

81. Chlamydia

Prevalence: 5.3 (per 1000 people in USA)

Chlamydia is a sexually transmitted diseased caused by the bacteria Chlamydia Trachomatis. Signs and symptoms include discharge, painful urination, pain during intercourse, discomfort, and few others. However, some individuals may never exhibit any symptoms. Although easily treatable with antibiotic therapy, serious complications can occur if left untreated. These complications can include Pelvic Inflammatory Disease, ectopic pregnancy, prostate infection, infertility, reactive arthritis, and several others. Proper management of Chlamydia is

Top 10 Foods: Chlamydia			
All Wild Caught/Organic/Grass-Fed/etc			
1	Garlic Cloves	6	Greek Yogurt
2	Echinacea	7	Black Beans
3	Goldenseal	8	Flaxseeds
4	Almonds	9	Chia Seeds
5	Walnuts	10	Kidney Beans

Bad Foods: Chlamydia	
Of the Foods Included in the Top 100	
Grass-Fed Beef	Red Wine

important to avoid these outcomes. Garlic, echinacea, and goldenseal are often considered for their potential antimicrobial and immune-boosting properties, which may be beneficial in supporting the body's natural defenses against infections like chlamydia.

82. Streptococcal Pharyngitis

Prevalence: 5.0 (per 1000 people in USA)

Streptococcal Pharyngitis (strep throat) is an upper respiratory bacterial infection that leads to sore throat, irritation, and phlegm formation. Other signs and symptoms include fever, chills, headache, red and swollen tonsils, body aches, and many more. Strep throat can cause extreme discomfort and impact quality of life during the course of the infection. Further, infection can spread to sinuses, tonsils, middle ear, and blood, resulting in more complications. Proper management and antibiotic therapy can help reduce symptoms and prevent spread of infection. Honey is often considered beneficial for

Top 10 Foods: Streptococcal Pharyngitis			
All Wild Caught/Organic/Grass-Fed/etc			
1	Local Honey	6	Pomegranates
2	Ginger Root	7	Strawberries
3	Eggs	8	Whole Oats
4	Turmeric Root	9	Blueberries
5	Chamomile Tea	10	Greek Yogurt

Bad Foods: Streptococcal Pharyngitis	
Of the Foods Included in the Top 100	
Lemons	Red Wine
Limes	Tomatoes

streptococcal pharyngitis due to its soothing properties and potential ability to help alleviate throat irritation and cough associated with the condition. Ginger root and turmeric root are believed to have anti-inflammatory and soothing properties.

83. Mononucleosis

Prevalence: 5.0 (per 1000 people in USA)

Infectious mononucleosis (mono) is a virus that is transmitted through saliva. Although usually associated with kissing, it can be spread by sharing drinking glass or utensils.

Although mono can have mild to no symptoms at times, serious complications such as an enlarged spleen or liver problems can occur. Usual signs and symptoms include fever, chills, fatigue, swollen lymph nodes, headache, swollen tonsils, and others. Proper management is important because mono can. decrease quality of life, performance, and impede day to day activities. Salmon,

Top 10 Foods: Mononucleosis			
All Wild Caught/Organic/Grass-Fed/etc			
1	Salmon	6	Green Tea
2	Mackerel	7	Spinach
3	Herring	8	Apples
4	Tomatoes	9	Kale
5	Bell Peppers	10	Chicken
Bad Foods: Mononucleosis			
Of the Foods Included in the Top 100			
Red Wine			

mackerel, and herring are beneficial for individuals with mononucleosis as they provide essential nutrients like omega-3 fatty acids and vitamin D, supporting immune function and overall health during the recovery from the infection. Tomatoes can be beneficial for individuals with mononucleosis as they are a rich source of vitamin C and antioxidants, potentially supporting immune function and aiding in the recovery process from the infection.

84. Hepatitis B

Prevalence: 4.6 (per 1000 people in USA)

Hepatitis B is a serious liver infection caused by the hepatitis B virus (HBV). Hepatitis B can result in serious problems such as liver failure, liver cirrhosis, and liver cancer. Hepatitis B

can cause a long list of symptoms, varying greatly in degree of severity. Hepatitis B can be transmitted through blood, semen, or bodily fluids. Transmission can often occur during sexual contact, sharing needles, accidental needle sticks, and from mother to child. Treatment and screening of Hepatitis B is very important to help control the spread and complications of Hepatitis B infection.

Top 10 Foods: Hepatitis B			
All Wild Caught/Organic/Grass-Fed/etc			
1	Extra Virgin Olive Oil	6	Spinach
2	Broccoli	7	Mackerel
3	Walnuts	8	Garlic Cloves
4	Avocados	9	Carrots
5	Salmon	10	Lemons
Bad Foods: Hepatitis B			
Of the Foods Included in the Top 100			
Red Wine			

Extra virgin olive oil may be beneficial for individuals with hepatitis B due to its anti-inflammatory properties and potential positive effects on liver health, supporting overall well-being in managing the infection.

85. Autism

Prevalence: 4.4 (per 1000 people in USA)

Autism spectrum disorder (Autism) is a medical condition associated with brain development resulting in unusual and different perceptions, social interactions, communication, ultimately affecting quality of life, daily activities, performance, and relationships. Boys are significantly more likely to develop Autism than girls. Proper management is critical in helping kids with Autism. Salmon, mackerel, and herring are considered beneficial for individuals with autism due to their rich content of omega-3 fatty acids, which may support cognitive function and neurological development.

Top 10 Foods: Autism			
All Wild Caught/Organic/Grass-Fed/etc			
1	Salmon	6	Sauerkraut
2	Mackerel	7	Seaweed
3	Herring	8	Kefir
4	Bananas	9	Chicken
5	Turkey	10	Lentils

Bad Foods: Autism	
Of the Foods Included in the Top 100	
Cheese	Milk
Greek Yogurt	

Including these fish in the diet can contribute to a nutrient-rich approach that may positively impact brain health and potentially alleviate some symptoms associated with autism spectrum disorders.

86. Rheumatoid Arthritis

Prevalence: 4.4 (per 1000 people in USA)

Rheumatoid Arthritis (RA) is a chronic, systemic, autoimmune, inflammatory disease that can affect multiple joints in the body along with damage to organs. Signs and symptoms include fatigue, stiff joints, painful joints, swollen joints, loss of appetite, and many more. When systemic, Rheumatoid Arthritis can impact skin, eyes, lungs, heart, and others. Rheumatoid Arthritis can significantly impact one's quality of life, daily activities,

Top 10 Foods: Rheumatoid Arthritis			
All Wild Caught/Organic/Grass-Fed/etc			
1	Salmon	6	Walnuts
2	Extra Virgin Olive Oil	7	Herring
3	Brown Rice	8	Quinoa
4	Mackerel	9	Turmeric Root
5	Whole Oats	10	Broccoli

and performance. Proper management is essential in controlling symptoms and complications from Rheumatoid Arthritis. Salmon, extra virgin olive oil, and brown rice are beneficial for individuals with rheumatoid arthritis as they collectively offer anti-inflammatory properties, omega-3 fatty acids, and whole-grain nutrients that may help manage inflammation and support joint health. Incorporating these foods into the diet can contribute to an arthritis-friendly approach, potentially easing symptoms and promoting overall well-being.

87. Cancer: Colon

Prevalence: 4.1 (per 1000 people in USA)

Colon cancer is a common cancer that starts in the large intestine (colon) of the digestive system. Even though Colon cancer normally begins in older adults, it can happen at any age. Initially, Colon cancer begins as benign polyps; those polyps can overtime become malignant. Signs and symptoms, although may be unnoticeable early on, include bowel movement changes, rectal bleedings, abdominal pain, weight loss, bloating, fatigue, and many others. Colon cancer can metastasize to other parts of the body at later stages. Prevention and proper

Top 10 Foods: Cancer: Colon			
All Wild Caught/Organic/Grass-Fed/etc			
1	Broccoli	6	Brown Rice
2	Salmon	7	Garlic Cloves
3	Mackerel	8	Lemons
4	Whole Oats	9	Herring
5	Oranges	10	Tomatoes

Bad Foods: Cancer: Colon	
Of the Foods Included in the Top 100	
Grass-Fed Beef	

management are critical. Broccoli, salmon, and whole oats are beneficial for individuals at risk of colon cancer as they provide a combination of fiber, omega-3 fatty acids, and antioxidants that support digestive health, reduce inflammation, and may contribute to the prevention of colon cancer. Including these foods in the diet promotes a colorectal-friendly approach, potentially reducing the risk and supporting overall colon health.

88. Raynaud's Syndrome

Prevalence: 4.0 (per 1000 people in USA)

Raynaud's mainly affects the fingers and toes of people with the disease, causing symptoms as a result of cold temperatures and stress. Raynaud's often affects the blood supply carried by smaller blood vessels, hence its effect on fingers and toes. Raynaud's is a vasospastic phenomena rather than a vaso-occlusive one. Symptoms of Raynaud's include: numbness, tingling, bluish/purple/red discoloration that can change to and from white and vice versa, aching and throbbing pain, and feeling cold to touch. Raynaud's

Top 10 Foods: Raynaud's Syndrome			
All Wild Caught/Organic/Grass-Fed/etc			
1	Salmon	6	Flaxseeds
2	Spinach	7	Chia Seeds
3	Almonds	8	Pumpkin Seeds
4	Walnuts	9	Ginkgo Biloba
5	Garlic Cloves	10	Strawberries

Disease can impact an individual's daily activity and quality of life. Several nutritional and dietary changes can help reduce signs and symptoms of Raynaud's. Salmon, spinach, and almonds are beneficial for individuals with Raynaud's syndrome as they contain nutrients like omega-3 fatty acids, vitamins, and minerals that may help improve blood circulation, reduce inflammation, and support vascular health, by promoting overall cardiovascular well-being and potentially alleviating episodes of cold-induced vasoconstriction.

89. Cancer: Skin / Melanoma

Prevalence: 3.7 (per 1000 people in USA)

Skin cancer is a common cancer affecting the skin when abnormal skin cells begin to grow and multiply. Often times, sun exposed areas are affected the most, and therefore, avoiding exposure to ultraviolet light (UV) can help prevent development of skin cancer. Areas most prone to sunlight include scalp, face, neck, arms, and few others. Types of skin cancer include basal cell carcinoma, melanoma, and squamous cell carcinoma. All

Top 10 Foods: Cancer: Skin / Melanoma			
All Wild Caught/Organic/Grass-Fed/etc			
1	Salmon	6	Broccoli
2	Spinach	7	Almonds
3	Kale	8	Oranges
4	Mackerel	9	Carrots
5	Herring	10	Lemons

types of skin cancer can metastasize to other parts of the body at later stages and if not managed properly. Salmon, mackerel, and herring are considered beneficial for individuals at risk of melanoma due to their rich omega-3 fatty acids content, which may have anti-inflammatory and protective effects on skin cells, potentially reducing the risk of melanoma development. Spinach and kale are beneficial for individuals at risk of melanoma due to their high levels of antioxidants, vitamins, and phytochemicals that may contribute to skin health and potentially offer protection against UV-induced damage.

90. HIV

Prevalence: 3.4 (per 1000 people in USA)

Human Immunodeficiency Virus (HIV) is a sexually transmitted disease that, if left untreated, can lead to Acquired Immunodeficiency Syndrome (AIDS). HIV is a virus that damages the immune system, resulting in weakened immunity and a significant decrease in the body's ability to fight off pathogens and diseases. Therefore, if not managed properly, HIV/AIDS can be life-threatening. Initially, when infected with HIV,

Top 10 Foods: HIV			
All Wild Caught/Organic/Grass-Fed/etc			
1	Broccoli	6	Ginger Root
2	Oranges	7	Brown Rice
3	Pineapple	8	Greek Yogurt
4	Spinach	9	Carrots
5	Apples	10	Avocados

flu like symptoms occur. Overtime, as the immune system weakens, exposure to serious opportunistic infections increases. Broccoli is considered beneficial for individuals with HIV due to its immune-boosting properties, providing essential nutrients and antioxidants that support overall immune function and potentially contribute to maintaining health in those living with HIV. Oranges and pineapple are beneficial for individuals with HIV as they are rich in vitamin C and antioxidants, potentially supporting immune function and overall health in individuals living with the virus.

91. Stroke / TIA

Prevalence: 3.4 (per 1000 people in USA)

Stroke is a serious problem that occurs when blood supply to the brain is diminished or disrupted. This results in decrease in oxygenation and nutrition to the brain, resulting in rapid death of brain cells. Signs and symptoms include paralysis, trouble speaking, trouble walking, face drooping and few others. A transient ischemic attack (TIA) is a very brief and mild stroke. Often times, TIA does not result in permanent damage. In both cases of stroke or TIA, Prevention and proper management are critical. Quality of life is significantly impacted in people that have a history of stroke. Salmon and mackerel are considered beneficial for stroke prevention due to their high omega-3 fatty acid content, which may contribute to maintaining cardiovascular health, reducing inflammation, and potentially lowering the risk of stroke. Whole oats and quinoa are beneficial for stroke prevention as they are rich in dietary fiber and essential nutrients, potentially aiding in managing blood pressure, and cholesterol levels.

Top 10 Foods: Stroke / TIA			
All Wild Caught/Organic/Grass-Fed/etc			
1	Salmon	6	Blueberries
2	Mackerel	7	Brown Rice
3	Whole Oats	8	Herring
4	Quinoa	9	Spinach
5	Strawberries	10	Broccoli

Bad Foods: Stroke / TIA
Of the Foods Included in the Top 100
Grass-Fed Beef

92. Shingles

Prevalence: 3.0 (per 1000 people in USA)

Shingles is a viral infection caused by varicella-zoster virus that results in an outbreak of painful rash and blisters. The virus that causes shingles is the same as chickenpox that has remained dormant in the individual's body and can become active during adulthood. Being over 50, immunocompromised, trauma, and stress can increase chances of getting Shingles. Besides excruciatingly painful rash and blisters, other symptoms can include fever, chills, fatigue, upset stomach, photosensitivity, headaches, and itching. Shingles can significantly affect an individual's daily activity and quality of life. Spinach is considered beneficial for individuals with shingles due to its high content of vitamins, minerals, and antioxidants, which may support immune function and overall well-being during the recovery from the viral infection.

Top 10 Foods: Shingles (Herpes Zoster)			
All Wild Caught/Organic/Grass-Fed/etc			
1	Spinach	6	Sardines
2	Salmon	7	Grass-Fed Beef
3	Kale	8	Chicken
4	Eggs	9	Bell Peppers
5	Carrots	10	

Bad Foods: Shingles (Herpes Zoster)	
Of the Foods Included in the Top 100	
Dark Chocolate	Red Wine

93. Multiple Sclerosis

Prevalence: 3.0 (per 1000 people in USA)

Multiple Sclerosis (MS) is an autoimmune disease of the central nervous system disease that results from the immune system attacking the protective sheath (myelin) that covers nerve fibers and causes communication problems between the brain and the rest of the body. Signs and symptoms include difficulty with walking, balance, and coordination, numbness, weakness, tremors and many others. There is no cure for MS, but proper management can help control symptoms and reduce severity. MS can drastically decrease quality of life,

Top 10 Foods: Multiple Sclerosis			
All Wild Caught/Organic/Grass-Fed/etc			
1	Salmon	6	Broccoli
2	Mackerel	7	Whole Oats
3	Herring	8	Oranges
4	Spinach	9	Walnuts
5	Kale	10	Garlic Cloves

Bad Foods: Multiple Sclerosis	
Of the Foods Included in the Top 100	
Grass-Fed Beef	

performance, and impede day to day activities. Salmon, mackerel, and herring are beneficial for individuals with multiple sclerosis due to their high omega-3 fatty acid content, which may have anti-inflammatory properties and support overall brain health, potentially contributing to the management of symptoms associated with the condition. Including these fatty fish in the diet will have protective effects on the nervous system.

94. Parkinson's

Prevalence: 3.0 (per 1000 people in USA)

Parkinson's disease is a progressive nervous system disorder that results in tremors, difficulty speaking, stiffness, and trouble with walking, balance, and coordination. Early on, signs and symptoms of Parkinson's disease can go unnoticed, but overtime, it can progress significantly and relatively quickly. There is no cure to Parkinson's disease, but proper management can help control symptoms and reduce severity. This is very

Top 10 Foods: Parkinson's			
All Wild Caught/Organic/Grass-Fed/etc			
1	Salmon	6	Blueberries
2	Mackerel	7	Walnuts
3	Herring	8	Tuna
4	Green Tea	9	Strawberries
5	Whole Oats	10	Brown Rice

important because Parkinson's disease can drastically decrease quality of life, performance, and impede day to day activities. Salmon, mackerel, and herring are considered beneficial for individuals with Parkinson's disease due to their rich omega-3 fatty acid content, which may possess neuroprotective properties and support brain health. The anti-inflammatory effects of these fatty fish may contribute to managing symptoms and potentially slowing the progression of Parkinson's disease.

95. Cancer: Thyroid
Prevalence: 2.5 (per 1000 people in USA)

Thyroid cancer is when cells in the thyroid gland become cancerous. The thyroid gland normally produces hormones that regulate your heart rate, blood pressure, body temperature and weight. Early on, thyroid cancer may go unnoticed, but over time the gland can become swollen and painful. Signs and symptoms include changes in voice, swollen lump in neck, trouble swallowing, swollen lymph nodes, and others. Thyroid cancer tends to have a higher occurrence in women than men. Prevention and proper management are critical. Brazil nuts are beneficial for individuals with thyroid cancer as they are an excellent source of selenium, a mineral known for its potential role in supporting thyroid function and aiding in the management of thyroid-related conditions.

Top 10 Foods: Cancer: Thyroid			
All Wild Caught/Organic/Grass-Fed/etc			
1	Brazil Nuts	6	Tuna
2	Chicken	7	Eggs
3	Greek Yogurt	8	Milk
4	Grass-Fed Beef	9	Oysters
5	Seaweed	10	Whole Oats

Bad Foods: Cancer: Thyroid	
Of the Foods Included in the Top 100	
Brussel Sprouts	Collard Greens
Cabbage	Soybeans

96. Cancer: Uterus / Endometrial
Prevalence: 2.4 (per 1000 people in USA)

Endometrial cancer is a type of cancer that begins in the layer of cells that form the lining (endometrium) of the uterus. The uterus is the hollow, pear-shaped pelvic organ where fetal development occurs. Endometrial cancer is often detected at an early stage because it frequently produces abnormal menstruation, post-menopausal bleeding, abnormal vaginal bleeding, and pelvic pain. If detected early, surgical removal of the uterus can be considered a cure. Early detection, prevention, and proper management are critical.

Top 10 Foods: Cancer: Uterus / Endometrial			
All Wild Caught/Organic/Grass-Fed/etc			
1	Salmon	6	Walnuts
2	Spinach	7	Herring
3	Kale	8	Raspberries
4	Mackerel	9	Broccoli
5	Almonds	10	Strawberries

Bad Foods: Cancer: Uterus / Endometrial	
Of the Foods Included in the Top 100	
Grass-Fed Beef	Red Wine

Salmon, spinach, and almonds are considered beneficial for individuals at risk of uterine cancer due to their combination of omega-3 fatty acids, vitamins, and antioxidants, which may have anti-inflammatory and protective effects that support overall reproductive health and potentially reduce the risk of uterine cancer. Including these foods in the diet can contribute to a well-rounded approach to promoting uterine health and supporting cancer prevention.

97. Cancer: Bladder

Prevalence: 2.2 (per 1000 people in USA)

Bladder cancer is a common type of cancer that begins in the cells (urothelial cells) that line the inside of the bladder, which is a hollow muscular organ in the lower abdomen that stores urine. Signs and symptoms include blood in urine, painful urination, frequent urination, and many others. Often times, bladder cancer can be detected at an early stage, making it easily treatable. However, bladder cancer can return and, therefore,

Top 10 Foods: Cancer: Bladder			
All Wild Caught/Organic/Grass-Fed/etc			
1	Kale	6	Spinach
2	Broccoli	7	Blueberries
3	Almonds	8	Oranges
4	Sweet Potatoes	9	Walnuts
5	Cauliflower	10	Garlic Cloves

follow-up testing is very important for years after successful treatment. Early detection, prevention, and proper management are critical. Kale, almonds, and sweet potatoes are beneficial for individuals at risk of bladder cancer as they provide a range of nutrients, including vitamins, antioxidants, and fiber, that may contribute to maintaining urinary tract health, reducing inflammation, and potentially lowering the risk of bladder cancer.

98. Cancer: Non-Hodgkin's Lymphoma

Prevalence: 2.2 (per 1000 people in USA)

Non-Hodgkin's lymphoma is cancer that originates in the lymphatic system, where tumors develop from a type of white blood cells called lymphocytes. The lymphatic system is the defense network spread throughout the body and, therefore, Non-Hodgkin's lymphoma can easily metastasize to nearly any tissue or organ in the body if not detected and treated early. Signs and symptoms of Non-Hodgkin's lymphoma include swollen and painful lymph nodes, fatigue, fever, weight loss, and many more. Early detection, prevention, and proper management are critical. Broccoli and salmon are beneficial for

Top 10 Foods: Cancer: Non-Hodgkin's Lymphoma			
All Wild Caught/Organic/Grass-Fed/etc			
1	Broccoli	6	Herring
2	Salmon	7	Collard Greens
3	Kale	8	Brussel Sprouts
4	Mackerel	9	Cauliflower
5	Walnuts	10	Spinach

Bad Foods: Cancer: Non-Hodgkin's Lymphoma	
Of the Foods Included in the Top 100	
Cheese	Greek Yogurt
Eggs	Milk
Grass-Fed Beef	

individuals with non-Hodgkin's lymphoma due to their anti-inflammatory properties, high content of antioxidants, and omega-3 fatty acids, which collectively may support immune function and potentially contribute to managing inflammation associated with the condition. Including these foods in the diet can be part of a comprehensive approach to supporting overall health in individuals with non-Hodgkin's lymphoma.

99. Brain Tumors

Prevalence: 2.1 (per 1000 people in USA)

A brain tumor is a growth or mass of abnormal cells in the brain. Several types of brain tumors exist, ranging from benign to malignant. Brain tumors can also be a result of metastasis from cancer in another part of the body. Signs and symptoms include headaches, fatigue, nausea/vomiting, speech difficulties, visual abnormalities, seizures, hearing problems, difficulty with balance and coordination, and many more. Brain tumors

Top 10 Foods: Brain Tumors			
All Wild Caught/Organic/Grass-Fed/etc			
1	Tomatoes	6	Sweet Potatoes
2	Broccoli	7	Raspberries
3	Brown Rice	8	Onions
4	Garlic Cloves	9	Quinoa
5	Carrots	10	Cauliflower

can have a significant impact on daily activities, performance, and quality of life. Early detection, prevention, and proper management are critical. Tomatoes are beneficial for individuals with brain tumors as they contain lycopene, an antioxidant that may have neuroprotective properties, potentially contributing to the overall health of the brain. The anti-inflammatory effects of lycopene, along with other nutrients in tomatoes, may support brain health and contribute to a well-rounded diet for those managing or preventing brain tumors.

100. Cardiomyopathy

Prevalence: 2.0 (per 1000 people in USA)

Cardiomyopathy is a pathologic heart muscle that results in difficulty for the heart to pump blood to the rest of the body. Cardiomyopathy can eventually lead to heart failure. Severity of cardiomyopathy can vary based on the three major types: dilated, hypertrophic, and restrictive. Signs and symptoms include fatigue, shortness of breath, swelling, chest discomfort, dizziness, and many others. Cardiomyopathy can have a significant

Top 10 Foods: Cardiomyopathy			
All Wild Caught/Organic/Grass-Fed/etc			
1	Salmon	6	Almonds
2	Mackerel	7	Whole Oats
3	Walnuts	8	Extra Virgin Olive Oil
4	Herring	9	Flaxseeds
5	Spinach	10	Kale

impact on daily activities, performance, and quality of life. Early detection, prevention, and proper management are critical. Salmon, mackerel, and herring are beneficial for individuals with cardiomyopathy due to their high omega-3 fatty acid content, which may support heart health by reducing inflammation, improving cardiac function, and potentially slowing the progression of cardiomyopathy. Including these fatty fish in the diet can be part of a heart-healthy approach that supports individuals managing this condition.

CHAPTER 4 – Top 100 Foods Ranked

Once we completed the Top 100 Diseases and Conditions, and the Top 10 for each one, we wanted to do a ranking of the Top 100 Foods. The proper statistical technique for something like this is called a "Nonparametric ranking".

This starts with a list of all the foods that were listed as good foods for each disease. This list could have been 10 foods long, or even 100 foods long (we only listed the top 10 for this book). Each food would have a number associated with it, telling us how many studies included that food for that disease. We took the metric for each food, and multiplied it by the prevalence of the disease out of one thousand. By summing all of these products, we would get what we call a weighted value for each food for one disease. Do this 100 times, and we have thousands of values. By summing all these numbers by the food, we would get a large list of foods with an overally ranking number. We ordered that number large to small, and standardized the highest number to 100 (the highest number would be the best food across all diseases. When we were completed, we actually had a list of 455 different foods, ranked 1 to 455. But we were only interested in the top 100.

If we let:
     P = Prevalence
     b = Disease/Condition
     a = food
     r = Rank of Food within a disease
     R = Total Rank of food

     Then
$$R_a = \sum (P_b * r_b) \text{ for } b = 1\text{-}100 \text{ for food } a$$

Do this for all foods, and we get 455 foods with a value of Ra for each. We take the top 100 in descending order, standardize the top food at a high of 100, and standardize the rest of the foods. We then have our Top 100 Foods.

So to make it more understandable:

"we ranked all 455 foods (identified in over 60,000 studies we looked at), based on the prevalence of the 100 diseases they were said to be good for, and took the top 100 of them for the book."

Top 100 Foods (Nonparametric Ranking)

#	Food	Score	#	Food	Score	#	Food	Score	#	Food	Score
1	Water	100.0	26	Sweet Potatoes	24.6	51	Cantaloupe	12.6	76	Green Beans	6.2
2	Salmon	68.0	27	Tomatoes	23.3	52	Green Tea	12.4	77	Cranberries	6.1
3	Spinach	49.5	28	Sardines	22.5	53	Pumpkin Seeds	12.1	78	Sunflower Seeds	5.7
4	Apples	44.4	29	Grapefruit	21.6	54	Squash	11.3	79	Chamomile Tea	5.0
5	Kale	40.8	30	Black Beans	20.7	55	Sauerkraut	11.1	80	Cucumbers	5.0
6	Mackerel	38.6	31	Raspberries	20.4	56	Seaweed	10.8	81	Celery	4.8
7	Broccoli	37.6	32	Flaxseeds	20.4	57	Potatoes	10.2	82	Peanuts	4.7
8	Chicken	36.1	33	Chia Seeds	19.2	58	Pineapple	9.7	83	Soybeans	4.3
9	Strawberries	35.7	34	Lentils	19.1	59	Whole Wheat	9.5	84	Mustard Greens	4.3
10	Almonds	35.7	35	Kidney Beans	18.9	60	Turmeric Root	9.0	85	Asparagus	4.2
11	Whole Oats	35.2	36	Collard Greens	18.1	61	Barley	8.8	86	Red Wine	4.0
12	Ginger Root	33.2	37	Chickpeas	17.2	62	Brussel Sprouts	8.6	87	Turnip Greens	3.5
13	Eggs	31.6	38	Milk	16.7	63	Pears	8.1	88	Buckwheat	3.4
14	Oranges	30.8	39	Onions	16.3	64	Beets	8.1	89	Bok Choy	3.2
15	Blueberries	30.8	40	Swiss Chard	16.1	65	Cauliflower	8.0	90	Mushrooms	3.1
16	Brown Rice	30.7	41	Cheese	16.1	66	Pistachios	7.6	91	Chili Peppers	3.1
17	Walnuts	29.5	42	Dark Chocolate	15.9	67	Kefir	7.4	92	Apricots	3.0
18	Greek Yogurt	28.6	43	Grass-Fed Beef	15.7	68	Tuna	7.1	93	Oysters	3.0
19	Garlic Cloves	28.4	44	Local Honey	14.5	69	Peas	6.9	94	Cashews	2.5
20	Carrots	28.0	45	Quinoa	14.5	70	Prunes	6.9	95	Mangoes	2.2
21	Avocados	26.0	46	Turkey	14.3	71	Kiwi	6.7	96	Eggplant	1.9
22	Bananas	25.7	47	Bell Peppers	14.1	72	Coconut Oil	6.6	97	Beef Liver	1.8
23	Lemons	25.5	48	Cherries	14.0	73	Grapes	6.5	98	Amaranth	0.6
24	Herring	25.4	49	Limes	13.4	74	Lettuce	6.3	99	Brazil Nuts	0.5
25	Extra Virgin Olive Oil	24.7	50	Cabbage	13.1	75	Apple Cider Vinegar	6.2	100	Pomegranates	0.3

And you see that each food in the top 100 has a number associated with it, that describes how it compares to the other 99 foods. But don't underestimate Pomegranates just because it is at #100 and scored 0.3, it is still a very powerful food, especially for in this case Streptococcal Pharyngitis.

Interestingly, if you counted up all the unique foods in the Top 10 across all diseases, we would end up with 104 unique foods, as there were 4 foods that while they were listed as a top 10, did not make the top 100. These foods were Ginkgo Biloba (Vertigo #1 and Raynaud's Syndrome #9), Fennel (Gerd #7), Echinacea (Chlamydia #2), and Goldenseal (Chlamydia #3). So while these 4 foods showed up in various Top 10's, they did not make the top 100.

We now present the "Top 100 Foods to Fight the Top 100 Diseases and Conditions in the United States".

1. Water

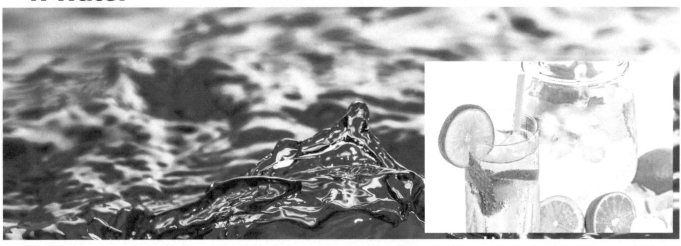

What is Water?

Water is a transparent, odorless, tasteless liquid that is essential for life. As we started researching all the best foods for the Top 100 Diseases, we quickly realized that is was listed in almost all studies as being very important. Originally, we did not plan on making it a "food", but the research was so convincing on its affect on human health that we included it in the Top 100.

Water is crucial for maintaining proper hydration, which is essential for bodily functions, including digestion, circulation, and temperature regulation. Water is a major component of cells and tissues. It helps transport nutrients and oxygen to cells and removes waste products. Water helps regulate body temperature through sweating and respiration. Drinking water aids digestion and helps prevent constipation by keeping the digestive tract lubricated. Water is a key component of synovial fluid, which lubricates and cushions joints. Water aids in the removal of waste products from the body and helps prevent all diseases associated with organs. Adequate water intake varies based on factors like age, gender, activity level, and climate.

Generally, it's recommended to drink about half of your body weight (in lbs) of water a day (in oz), though individual needs may vary (for example, if a person weighs 150 lbs, they should drink 75 oz a day).

Top Diseases/Conditions

Water is identified as a top food for all 100 of the Top 100 Diseases and Conditions. Of those, all Diseases and Conditions rank it as #1 (Golden Bullets)!

100 Golden Bullets		Definition: #1 Top Food for each given condition
Acne	COPD	Mononucleosis
ADHD	Coronary Artery Disease	Multiple Sclerosis
Allergies Rhinitis	Depression	Obesity
Alopecia Areata	Diverticulitis	OCD
Alzheimer's/Dementia	Endometriosis	Oral/Dental Health
Anemia of Chronic Disease	Epilepsy	Osteoarthritis
Anxiety Disorder	Fibroids	Osteoporosis
Aortic Aneurysm	Fibromyalgia	Parkinson's
Arrhythmia	Gallstone	Pelvic Inflammatory Disease
Asthma	Gastritis	Peptic Ulcer
Atopic Dermatitis	Gastroenteritis	Peripheral Arterial Disease
Autism	Genital Herpes	Plantar Warts
Bipolar Disorder	GERD/Heartburn	Pneumonia
Brain Tumors	Glaucoma	Pregnancy
C: Non-Hodgkin's Lymphoma	Gout	Premenstrual Syndrome
Cancer: Bladder	Heart Failure	Psoriasis
Cancer: Breast	Hemorrhoids	Raynaud's Syndrome
Cancer: Colon	Hepatitis B	Rheumatoid Arthritis
Cancer: Prostate	Hepatitis C	Rosacea
Cancer: Skin/Melanoma	High Cholesterol	Schizophrenia
Cancer: Thyroid	HIV	Shingles
Cancer: Uterus/Endometrial	Hypertension	Sleep Apnea
Cardiomyopathy	Hyperthyroidism	Streptococcal Pharyngitis
Cataracts	Hypothyroidism	Stroke/TIA
Celiac Disease	Inflammatory Bowel Disease	Syncope
Chlamydia	Influenza	Tinnitus
Chronic Kidney Disease	Inguinal Hernia	Tuberculosis
Chronic Liver Disease	Insomnia	Type I Diabetes
Cold Sores	Iron Deficiency Anemia	Type II Diabetes
Common Cold/Virus	Irritable Bowel Syndrome	Urinary Tract Infection
Congenital Heart Defect	Kidney Stone	Valvular Heart Disease
Conjunctivitis	Lumbar Radiculopathy	Vertigo
Constipation	Menopause	
Contact Dermatitis	Migraine	

2. Salmon

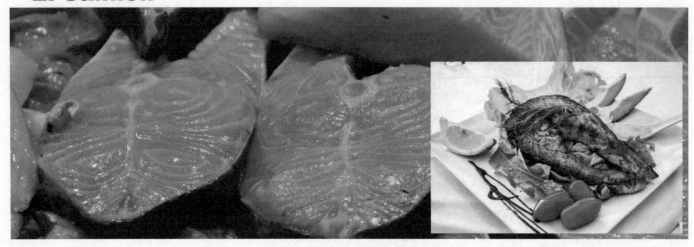

What is Salmon?

Salmon is a nutrient-rich fish renowned for its distinctive flavor, tender flesh, and numerous health benefits. This fatty fish belongs to the family Salmonidae and is found in both saltwater and freshwater environments. Salmon is prized for its exceptional omega-3 fatty acid content, particularly eicosapentaenoic acid (EPA) and docosahexaenoic acid (DHA), which are crucial for heart health, brain function, and reducing inflammation in the body.

In addition to omega-3s, salmon is an excellent source of high-quality protein, essential vitamins, and minerals. It provides a wealth of nutrients such as vitamin B12, vitamin D, selenium, and iodine, contributing to overall well-being. The pink or reddish color of salmon flesh is attributed to natural pigments like astaxanthin, which also acts as a potent antioxidant.

Whether grilled, baked, smoked, or raw in sushi, salmon's versatility in the kitchen makes it a popular and nutritious choice, promoting cardiovascular health, supporting brain function, and offering a delectable addition to a balanced diet.

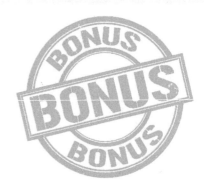

Top 6 Salmon		
	All Wild Caught	Omega-3 (DHA+EPA)
	Type (85g Serving)	mg
1	King Chinook (Pacific)	1638 (328% DRI)
2	Atlantic (Atlantic)	1206 (241%)
3	Sockeye (Pacific)	984 (197%)
4	Coho (Pacific)	912 (182%)
5	Pink (Pacific)	843 (169%)
6	Chum (Pacific)	525 (105%)

Top Diseases/Conditions

Salmon is identified as a top food for 86 of the Top 100 Diseases and Conditions. Of those, 40 Diseases and Conditions rank it as #1 (Golden Bullets), while 39 of them rank it between #2 and #10 (Silver Bullets).

40 Golden Bullets	Definition: #1 Top Food for each given condition (other than Water)
Acne	Heart Failure
ADHD	High Cholesterol
Allergies Rhinitis	Hypertension
Alopecia Areata	Irritable Bowel Syndrome (IBS)
Arrhythmia / Afib	Menopause
Atopic Dermatitis	Migrain
Autism	Mononucleosis
Bipolar Disorder	Multiple Sclerosis
Cancer: Skin / Melanoma	Osteoarthritis
Cancer: Uterus / Endometrial	Osteoporosis
Cardiomyopathy	Parkinson's
Cataracts	Pelvic Inflammatory Disease
Cold Sores	Peptic Ulcer
Congenital Heart Defect	Premenstrual Syndrome
Contact Dermatitis	Psoriasis
COPD	Raynaud's Syndrome
Coronary Artery Disease	Rheumatoid Arthritis
Endometriosis	Schizophrenia
Fibromyalgia	Stroke / TIA
Genital Herpes	Valvular Heart Disease

39 Silver Bullets	Definition: Top 10 food for each given condition (but not #1)
Alzheimer's / Dementia	Hyperthyroidism
Anxiety Disorder	Inflammatory Bowel Disease
Aortic Aneurysm	Influenza
Asthma	Insomnia
Cancer: Breast	Lumbar Radiculopathy
Cancer: Colon	Obesity
Cancer: Non-Hodgkin's Lymphoma	OCD
Cancer: Prostate	Peripheral Artery Disease
Chronic Kidney Disease	Pneumonia
Chronic Liver Disease	Pregnancy
Common Cold / Virus	Rosacea
Depression	Shingles (Herpes Zoster)
Fibroids	Sleep Apnea
Gallstones	Syncope
Gastritis	Tuberculosis (TB)
Gastroenteritis	Type I Diabetes
Glaucoma	Type II Diabetes
Gout	Urinary Tract Infection
Hepatitis B	Vertigo
Hepatitis C	

Nutrients?

One serving (85g, 121 Calories) of Wild-Caught Atlantic Salmon contains:

14 Significant Nutrients

Nutrient	DRI Per Serving (Daily Recommended Intake)
Omega-3 DHA	379%
Vitamin B12	113%
Omega-3 EPA	109%
Selenium	56%
Vitamin B6	53%
Vitamin B3 (Niacin)	42%
Protein	30%
Vitamin B5 (Pantothenic Acid)	28%
Vitamin B2 (Riboflavin)	26%
Phosphorus	24%
Copper	24%
Vitamin B7 (Biotin)	17%
Vitamin B1 (Thiamine)	14%
Potassium	12%

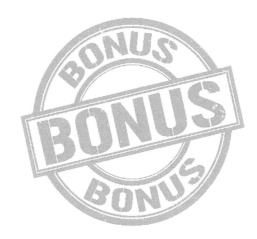

Top Seafood

Type	Calories	Percent DRI per serving				
		Omega-3 DHA	Omega-3 EPA	Zinc	B12	Copper
Salmon	121	379%	109%	< 10%	113%	24%
Mackeral	174	476%	305%	< 10%	308%	11%
Sardines	177	173%	161%	10%	316%	19%
Herring	134	293%	241%	< 10%	483%	11%
Oysters	58	99%	91%	701%	690%	419%
Tuna	109	214%	79%	< 10%	42%	< 10%

Best   2nd Best

3. Spinach

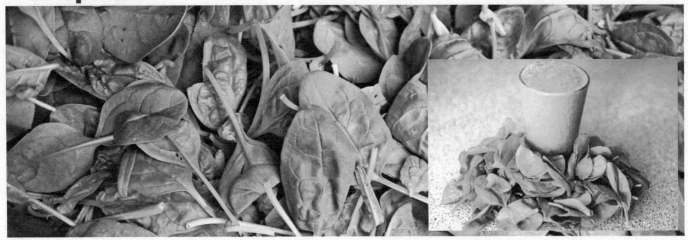

What is Spinach?

Spinach, a verdant leafy green, is a nutritional powerhouse with a wealth of health benefits. Rich in essential vitamins and minerals, spinach is particularly notable for its high content of vitamin K, crucial for blood clotting and bone health. A single cup of cooked spinach can provide well over the recommended daily intake of vitamin K, supporting overall cardiovascular and skeletal well-being.

Additionally, spinach is an excellent source of vitamin A, in the form of beta-carotene. This antioxidant plays a pivotal role in maintaining healthy skin, promoting vision, and supporting immune function. Regular consumption of spinach contributes not only to meeting vitamin requirements but also provides a host of other nutrients, including iron, folate, and fiber. Whether incorporated into salads, sautéed, or blended into smoothies, spinach stands out as a versatile and nutritious addition to a balanced diet, fostering overall health and vitality.

Top Diseases/Conditions

Spinach is identified as a top food for 74 of the Top 100 Diseases and Conditions. Of those, 22 Diseases and Conditions rank it as #1 (Golden Bullets), while 34 of them rank it between #2 and #10 (Silver Bullets).

22 Golden Bullets	Definition: #1 Top Food for each given condition (other than Water)
Alzheimer's / Dementia	Iron Deficiency Anemia
Anemia of Chronic Disease	Lumbar Radiculopathy
Asthma	Migrain
Cancer: Skin / Melanoma	Oral / Dental Health
Cancer: Uterus / Endometrial	Osteoarthritis
Cataracts	Pelvic Inflammatory Disease
Conjunctivitis	Plantar Warts
Constipation	Psoriasis
Fibromyalgia	Shingles (Herpes Zoster)
Gallstones	Syncope
Hypertension	Tinnitus

34 Silver Bullets	Definition: Top 10 food for each given condition (but not #1)
Acne	Hepatitis C
ADHD	HIV
Alopecia Areata	Hyperthyroidism
Anxiety Disorder	Inguinal Hernia
Bipolar Disorder	Mononucleosis
Cancer: Bladder	Multiple Sclerosis
Cancer: Non-Hodgkin's Lymphoma	OCD
Cardiomyopathy	Osteoporosis
Common Cold / Virus	Peripheral Artery Disease
Contact Dermatitis	Pregnancy
COPD	Premenstrual Syndrome
Depression	Raynaud's Syndrome
Endometriosis	Rosacea
Epilepsy	Schizophrenia
Fibroids	Stroke / TIA
Gastritis	Type I Diabetes
Hepatitis B	Type II Diabetes

Nutrients?

One serving (1 Cup, 30g, 7 Calories) contains:

5 Significant Nutrients	
Nutrient	DRI Per Serving (Daily Recommended Intake)
Vitamin K	121%
Vitamin A	94%
Vitamin B9 (Folate)	15%
Manganese	13%
Iron	10%

4. Apples

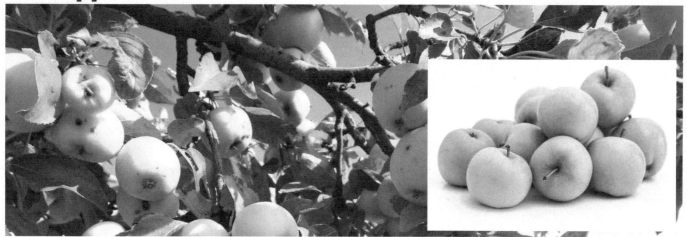

What are Apples?

Apples, scientifically known as Malus domestica, are popular fruits with a crisp texture and a sweet or tart flavor. These fruits are not only delicious but also packed with essential nutrients. Apples are a rich source of dietary fiber, particularly soluble fiber called pectin, which promotes digestive health, aids in weight management, and helps regulate blood sugar levels.

In addition to fiber, apples contain vitamin C, a potent antioxidant that supports the immune system, aids in collagen production for skin health, and acts as an overall cellular protector. Furthermore, apples provide trace amounts of copper, an essential mineral involved in various physiological processes, including iron metabolism and the formation of connective tissues.

Whether enjoyed fresh, sliced into salads, or transformed into applesauce, the nutritional profile of apples makes them a smart choice for a healthy, balanced diet, contributing to overall well-being and offering a deliciously crunchy snack.

The antioxidant content in apples can vary depending on the variety. Two of the apple varieties known for their high antioxidant content are Granny Smith and Red Delicious.

Top Diseases/Conditions

Apples are identified as a top food for 31 of the Top 100 Diseases and Conditions. Of those, 4 Diseases and Conditions rank it as #1 (Golden Bullets), while 18 of them rank it between #2 and #10 (Silver Bullets).

4 Golden Bullets	Definition: #1 Top Food for each given condition (other than Water)
Aortic Aneurysm	Diverticulitis
Constipation	Gastroenteritis

18 Silver Bullets	Definition: Top 10 food for each given condition (but not #1)
Asthma	HIV
Atopic Dermatitis	Hypertension
Chronic Kidney Disease	Inguinal Hernia
Cold Sores	Mononucleosis
Common Cold / Virus	Oral / Dental Health
Gastritis	Peripheral Artery Disease
Genital Herpes	Plantar Warts
Hemorrhoids	Schizophrenia
High Cholesterol	Sleep Apnea

Nutrients?

One serving (1 Apple, 242g, 126 Calories) of a Granny Smith Apple contains:

3 Significant Nutrients	
Nutrient	DRI Per Serving (Daily Recommended Intake)
Fiber	15%
Vitamin C	12%
Copper	11%

5. Kale

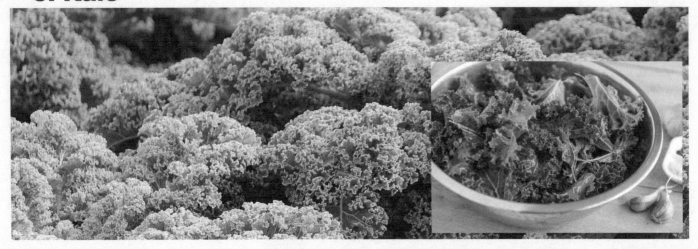

What is Kale?

Kale, a leafy green vegetable belonging to the Brassicaceae family, is celebrated for its robust nutritional profile and versatile culinary applications. Packed with vitamins and minerals, kale is a standout choice for promoting overall health. Notably, kale is exceptionally rich in vitamin K, crucial for blood clotting, bone metabolism, and cardiovascular health.

Moreover, kale is a potent source of vitamin A, derived from beta-carotene, promoting eye health, immune function, and skin integrity. Additionally, kale provides a significant dose of vitamin C, a powerful antioxidant known for supporting immune function, collagen synthesis, and overall cellular protection.

This nutrient-dense green can be enjoyed raw in salads, blended into smoothies, or lightly cooked, offering a delicious and healthful addition to a well-rounded diet. Incorporating kale into meals provides a spectrum of essential nutrients, contributing to overall well-being and vitality.

Top Diseases/Conditions

Kale is identified as a top food for 68 of the Top 100 Diseases and Conditions. Of those, 15 Diseases and Conditions rank it as #1 (Golden Bullets), while 35 of them rank it between #2 and #10 (Silver Bullets).

15 Golden Bullets	Definition: #1 Top Food for each given condition (other than Water)
Asthma	Hypertension
Cancer: Bladder	Kidney Stone
Cancer: Breast	Lumbar Radiculopathy
Cancer: Skin / Melanoma	Oral / Dental Health
Cancer: Uterus / Endometrial	Osteoporosis
Fibromyalgia	Pregnancy
Gallstones	Psoriasis
Hepatitis C	

35 Silver Bullets	Definition: Top 10 food for each given condition (but not #1)
Acne	Influenza
Alzheimer's / Dementia	Inguinal Hernia
Anemia of Chronic Disease	Iron Deficiency Anemia
Arrhythmia / Afib	Migrain
Cancer: Non-Hodgkin's Lymphoma	Mononucleosis
Cardiomyopathy	Multiple Sclerosis
Common Cold / Virus	Osteoarthritis
Congenital Heart Defect	Peripheral Artery Disease
Conjunctivitis	Plantar Warts
Contact Dermatitis	Pneumonia
COPD	Premenstrual Syndrome
Coronary Artery Disease	Schizophrenia
Endometriosis	Shingles (Herpes Zoster)
Epilepsy	Sleep Apnea
Fibroids	Tinnitus
Glaucoma	Type I Diabetes
Heart Failure	Valvular Heart Disease
Hyperthyroidism	

Nutrients?

One serving (1 Cup, 67g, 34 Calories) contains:

7 Significant Nutrients	
Nutrient	DRI Per Serving (Daily Recommended Intake)
Vitamin K	456%
Vitamin A	343%
Vitamin C	89%
Copper	22%
Manganese	22%
Vitamin B6	15%
Iron	14%

6. Mackerel

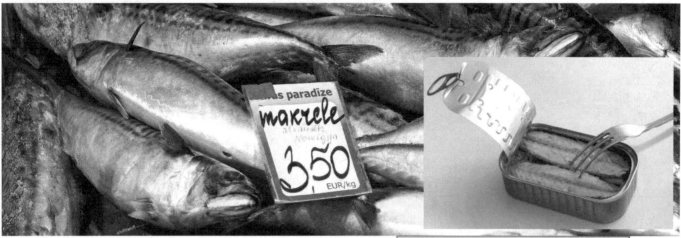

What is Mackerel?

Mackerel, a fatty fish belonging to the Scombridae family, is a nutrient-rich seafood known for its distinctive flavor and numerous health benefits. Rich in omega-3 fatty acids, mackerel is an excellent source of both docosahexaenoic acid (DHA) and eicosapentaenoic acid (EPA). These omega-3s play crucial roles in supporting cardiovascular health, brain function, and reducing inflammation throughout the body.

Furthermore, mackerel is a standout source of vitamin B12, essential for neurological function, DNA synthesis, and the formation of red blood cells. Adequate vitamin B12 intake is vital for overall energy metabolism and maintaining a healthy nervous system.

Incorporating mackerel into a balanced diet, whether grilled, baked, or canned, provides a flavorful way to obtain essential nutrients, supporting heart and brain health, and contributing to overall well-being.

Top Diseases/Conditions

Mackerel is identified as a top food for 67 of the Top 100 Diseases and Conditions. Of those, 20 Diseases and Conditions rank it as #1 (Golden Bullets), while 35 of them rank it between #2 and #10 (Silver Bullets).

20 Golden Bullets	Definition: #1 Top Food for each given condition (other than Water)
Alopecia Areata	Coronary Artery Disease
Arrhythmia / Afib	Endometriosis
Autism	Genital Herpes
Bipolar Disorder	Heart Failure
Cancer: Skin / Melanoma	Multiple Sclerosis
Cancer: Uterus / Endometrial	Parkinson's
Cardiomyopathy	Psoriasis
Cold Sores	Schizophrenia
Congenital Heart Defect	Stroke / TIA
Contact Dermatitis	Valvular Heart Disease

35 Silver Bullets	Definition: Top 10 food for each given condition (but not #1)
Acne	Hepatitis C
ADHD	High Cholesterol
Allergies Rhinitis	Inflammatory Bowel Disease
Alzheimer's / Dementia	Insomnia
Atopic Dermatitis	Irritable Bowel Syndrome (IBS)
Cancer: Breast	Menopause
Cancer: Colon	Migrain
Cancer: Non-Hodgkin's Lymphoma	Mononucleosis
Cancer: Prostate	OCD
Chronic Kidney Disease	Osteoarthritis
COPD	Pneumonia
Depression	Premenstrual Syndrome
Epilepsy	Rheumatoid Arthritis
Fibromyalgia	Tuberculosis (TB)
Gallstones	Type I Diabetes
Glaucoma	Type II Diabetes
Gout	Urinary Tract Infection
Hepatitis B	

Nutrients?

One serving (85g, 174 Calories) of Mackerel contains:

16 Significant Nutrients	
Nutrient	DRI Per Serving (Daily Recommended Intake)
Omega-3 DHA	476%
Vitamin B12	308%
Omega-3 EPA	305%
Selenium	68%
Vitamin D	51%
Vitamin B3 (Niacin)	48%
Protein	28%
Phosphorus	26%
Vitamin B6	23%
Vitamin B2 (Riboflavin)	23%
"Good" Fat	18%
Iron	18%
Magnesium	15%
Vitamin B5 (Pantothenic Acid)	14%
Copper	11%
Choline	10%

7. Broccoli

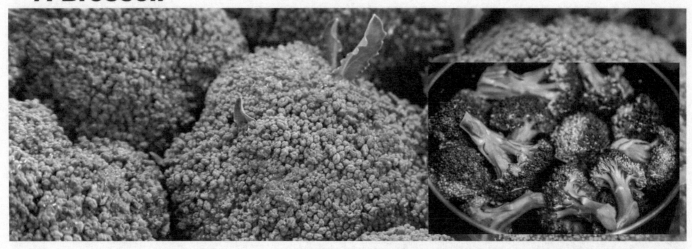

What is Broccoli?

Broccoli, a cruciferous vegetable in the Brassicaceae family, is celebrated for its nutritional density and versatile culinary applications. Rich in vitamins and minerals, broccoli is particularly notable for its high content of vitamin C, a powerful antioxidant that supports the immune system, promotes skin health, and aids in collagen synthesis.

Additionally, broccoli is a significant source of vitamin K, essential for blood clotting, bone metabolism, and cardiovascular health. This vitamin K content contributes to maintaining strong and healthy bones.

Whether steamed, sautéed, or enjoyed raw, broccoli is a valuable addition to a balanced diet, offering a spectrum of nutrients and potential health benefits. Incorporating broccoli into meals provides a delicious and nutritious way to support overall well-being, making it a versatile and health-conscious choice for a variety of culinary creations.

Top Diseases/Conditions

Broccoli is identified as a top food for 61 of the Top 100 Diseases and Conditions. Of those, 15 Diseases and Conditions rank it as #1 (Golden Bullets), while 36 of them rank it between #2 and #10 (Silver Bullets).

15 Golden Bullets	Definition: #1 Top Food for each given condition (other than Water)
Cancer: Bladder	Kidney Stone
Cancer: Colon	Lumbar Radiculopathy
Cancer: Non-Hodgkin's Lymphoma	Menopause
Chronic Liver Disease	Obesity
Constipation	Peptic Ulcer
Epilepsy	Peripheral Artery Disease
Fibroids	Psoriasis
HIV	

36 Silver Bullets	Definition: Top 10 food for each given condition (but not #1)
Alopecia Areata	Hepatitis B
Arrhythmia / Afib	Hepatitis C
Asthma	Inflammatory Bowel Disease
Brain Tumors	Influenza
Cancer: Breast	Iron Deficiency Anemia
Cancer: Prostate	Multiple Sclerosis
Cancer: Skin / Melanoma	Oral / Dental Health
Cancer: Uterus / Endometrial	Osteoarthritis
Cataracts	Plantar Warts
Celiac Disease	Pregnancy
Common Cold / Virus	Premenstrual Syndrome
Congenital Heart Defect	Rheumatoid Arthritis
Conjunctivitis	Schizophrenia
Contact Dermatitis	Sleep Apnea
Coronary Artery Disease	Stroke / TIA
Endometriosis	Tinnitus
Heart Failure	Type II Diabetes
Hemorrhoids	Valvular Heart Disease

Nutrients?

One serving (148g, 50 Calories) contains:

13 Significant Nutrients	
Nutrient	DRI Per Serving (Daily Recommended Intake)
Vitamin C	147%
Vitamin K	125%
Vitamin A	31%
Vitamin B9 (Folate)	23%
Vitamin B6	23%
Vitamin B5 (Pantothenic Acid)	16%
Vitamin B2 (Riboflavin)	15%
Phosphorus	14%
Potassium	14%
Iron	14%
Manganese	13%
Copper	11%
Fiber	10%

8. Chicken

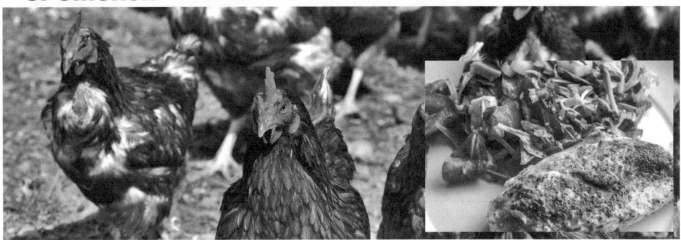

What is Chicken?

Chickens, domesticated fowl from the Gallus gallus species, are a widely consumed protein source with various cuts, and one popular choice is skinless chicken breast. Renowned for its lean profile, skinless chicken breast is an excellent source of high-quality protein, essential for muscle development, repair, and overall body function.

In addition to being a protein powerhouse, chicken breast contains vitamin B3, also known as niacin. Niacin is crucial for energy metabolism, supporting the nervous system, and promoting skin health. Consuming skinless chicken breast as part of a balanced diet provides essential nutrients while being low in saturated fat.

Whether grilled, baked, or sautéed, incorporating skinless chicken breast into meals offers a versatile and nutritious protein option, contributing to overall health and well-being. This lean meat is a staple in many diets worldwide, providing essential nutrients for maintaining a healthy and active lifestyle.

Top Diseases/Conditions

Chicken is identified as a top food for 44 of the Top 100 Diseases and Conditions. Of those, 1 Diseases and Conditions rank it as #1 (Golden Bullets), while 23 of them rank it between #2 and #10 (Silver Bullets).

1 Golden Bullet	Definition: #1 Top Food for each given condition (other than Water)
Kidney Stone	

23 Silver Bullets	Definition: Top 10 food for each given condition (but not #1)
ADHD	Hyperthyroidism
Alopecia Areata	Hypothyroidism
Anemia of Chronic Disease	Irritable Bowel Syndrome (IBS)
Autism	Migrain
Cancer: Thyroid	Mononucleosis
Celiac Disease	OCD
Cold Sores	Pregnancy
COPD	Schizophrenia
Gastroenteritis	Shingles (Herpes Zoster)
Genital Herpes	Tinnitus
GERD / Heartburn	Urinary Tract Infection
Gout	

Nutrients?

One serving (85g, 94 Calories) contains:

8 Significant Nutrients	
Nutrient	DRI Per Serving (Daily Recommended Intake)
Vitamin B3 (Niacin)	59%
Protein	35%
Vitamin B6	33%
Selenium	28%
Phosphorus	24%
Vitamin B5 (Pantothenic Acid)	14%
Vitamin B12	12%
Choline	11%

9. Strawberries

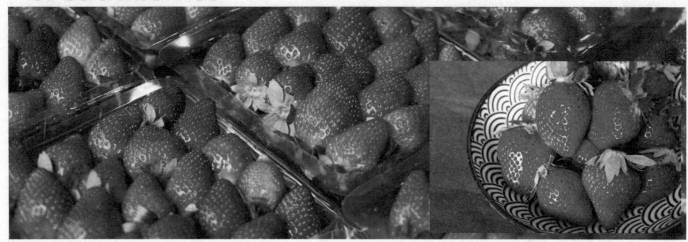

What are Strawberries?

Strawberries, fragrant berries from the Fragaria x ananassa plant, are not only delectably sweet but also brimming with nutritional benefits. Renowned for their vibrant red hue and succulent taste, strawberries are an excellent source of vitamin C, a powerful antioxidant crucial for immune system function, collagen synthesis, and overall cellular protection.

In addition to vitamin C, strawberries offer a spectrum of nutrients, including folate, manganese, and antioxidants like quercetin and anthocyanins. These compounds contribute to heart health, may help regulate blood sugar levels, and possess anti-inflammatory properties.

Whether enjoyed fresh on their own, added to salads, or blended into smoothies, strawberries make a delightful and healthful addition to a balanced diet. Their natural sweetness, combined with a wealth of nutrients, positions strawberries as a versatile and nutritious fruit that not only satisfies the taste buds but also supports overall well-being.

Top Diseases/Conditions

Strawberries are identified as a top food for 48 of the Top 100 Diseases and Conditions. Of those, 5 Diseases and Conditions rank it as #1 (Golden Bullets), while 21 of them rank it between #2 and #10 (Silver Bullets).

5 Golden Bullets	Definition: #1 Top Food for each given condition (other than Water)
Allergies Rhinitis	Hypertension
Alzheimer's/Dementia	Type I Diabetes
Epilepsy	

21 Silver Bullets	Definition: Top 10 food for each given condition (but not #1)
Cancer: Breast	Irritable Bowel Syndrome (IBS)
Cancer: Prostate	Parkinson's
Cancer: Uterus / Endometrial	Plantar Warts
Cataracts	Pneumonia
Chronic Kidney Disease	Psoriasis
Conjunctivitis	Raynaud's Syndrome
Endometriosis	Streptococcal Pharyngitis
Gastritis	Stroke / TIA
Gastroenteritis	Type II Diabetes
Hemorrhoids	Urinary Tract Infection
High Cholesterol	

Nutrients?

One serving (147g, 47 Calories) contains:

3 Significant Nutrients	
Nutrient	DRI Per Serving (Daily Recommended Intake)
Vitamin C	96%
Manganese	26%
Copper	11%

10. Almonds

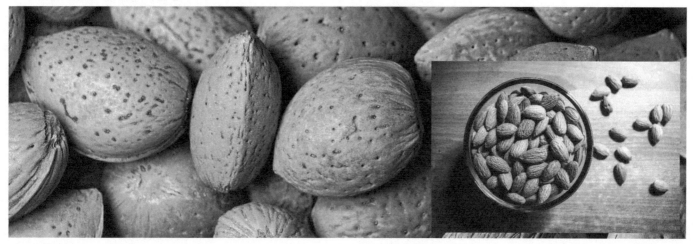

What are Almonds?

Almonds, the seeds of the Prunus dulcis tree, are nutrient-dense nuts renowned for their delightful taste and numerous health benefits. Rich in vitamin E, almonds are a powerful antioxidant that supports skin health, protects cells from oxidative stress, and contributes to overall immune function.

In addition to vitamin E, almonds provide essential minerals such as copper and manganese. Copper is vital for iron metabolism, connective tissue formation, and overall cardiovascular health, while manganese plays a role in bone development, blood clotting, and antioxidant enzyme function.

Whether eaten raw, roasted, or transformed into almond butter, almonds offer a delicious and versatile way to incorporate healthy fats, protein, and an array of nutrients into a balanced diet. Their crunchy texture and nutrient-rich profile make almonds a popular and health-conscious snack choice, contributing to overall well-being.

Top Diseases/Conditions

Almonds are identified as a top food for 65 of the Top 100 Diseases and Conditions. Of those, 14 Diseases and Conditions rank it as #1 (Golden Bullets), while 26 of them rank it between #2 and #10 (Silver Bullets).

14 Golden Bullets	Definition: #1 Top Food for each given condition (other than Water)
Arrhythmia / Afib	Heart Failure
Cancer: Bladder	High Cholesterol
Cancer: Uterus / Endometrial	Insomnia
Chronic Liver Disease	OCD
Congenital Heart Defect	Oral / Dental Health
Coronary Artery Disease	Pelvic Inflammatory Disease
Gout	Valvular Heart Disease

26 Silver Bullets	Definition: Top 10 food for each given condition (but not #1)
Acne	Fibromyalgia
Alopecia Areata	GERD / Heartburn
Alzheimer's / Dementia	Hepatitis C
Anxiety Disorder	Influenza
Aortic Aneurysm	Menopause
Cancer: Prostate	Obesity
Cancer: Skin / Melanoma	Osteoarthritis
Cardiomyopathy	Peripheral Artery Disease
Cataracts	Premenstrual Syndrome
Celiac Disease	Raynaud's Syndrome
Chlamydia	Schizophrenia
Endometriosis	Syncope
Epilepsy	Tinnitus

Nutrients?

One serving (28g, 167 Calories) contains:

10 Significant Nutrients	
Nutrient	DRI Per Serving (Daily Recommended Intake)
Vitamin E	49%
Copper	33%
Manganese	30%
"Good" Fat	27%
Omega 6 LA	21%
Phosphorus	20%
Magnesium	19%
Iron	16%
Vitamin B2 (Riboflavin)	15%
Protein	11%

11. Whole Oats

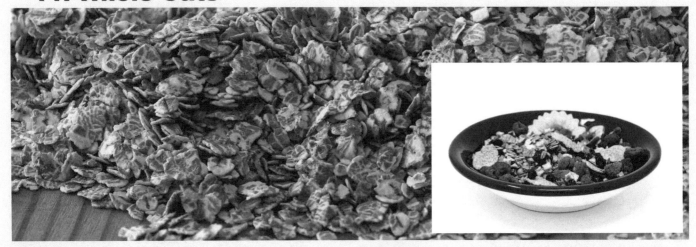

What are Whole Oats?

Whole oats, derived from the Avena sativa plant, are a nutritious and gluten-free cereal grain celebrated for their versatility and health benefits. Rich in manganese, whole oats support bone development, metabolism, and antioxidant enzyme function. Manganese also contributes to collagen formation and overall connective tissue health.

Whole oats are a good source of phosphorus, essential for bone and teeth formation, kidney function, and energy metabolism. These minerals make whole oats a nutrient-dense food.

Importantly, whole oats are naturally gluten-free, making them suitable for individuals with gluten sensitivities or celiac disease. This distinguishes them from other grains containing gluten, such as wheat, barley, and rye. Whether enjoyed as oatmeal, added to smoothies, or incorporated into gluten-free baked goods, whole oats provide a wholesome and nourishing option, supporting bone health, metabolism, and catering to dietary preferences for those seeking gluten-free alternatives.

Top Diseases/Conditions

WhOats are identified as a top food for 54 of the Top 100 Diseases and Conditions. Of those, 6 Diseases and Conditions rank it as #1 (Golden Bullets), while 29 of them rank it between #2 and #10 (Silver Bullets).

6 Golden Bullets	Definition: #1 Top Food for each given condition (other than Water)
GERD / Heartburn	Peptic Ulcer
Gout	Peripheral Artery Disease
High Cholesterol	Stroke / TIA

29 Silver Bullets	Definition: Top 10 food for each given condition (but not #1)
Anxiety Disorder	Inguinal Hernia
Atopic Dermatitis	Insomnia
Bipolar Disorder	Lumbar Radiculopathy
Cancer: Breast	Multiple Sclerosis
Cancer: Colon	Obesity
Cancer: Thyroid	OCD
Cardiomyopathy	Parkinson's
Constipation	Pregnancy
COPD	Rheumatoid Arthritis
Diverticulitis	Rosacea
Fibroids	Sleep Apnea
Gastroenteritis	Streptococcal Pharyngitis
Hemorrhoids	Type II Diabetes
Hepatitis C	Urinary Tract Infection
Inflammatory Bowel Disease	

Nutrients?

One serving (44g, 171 Calories) (Typical Serving is ½ Cup Cooked, 1/7 Cup Dry) contains:

11 Significant Nutrients	
Nutrient	DRI Per Serving (Daily Recommended Intake)
Manganese	94%
Phosphorus	33%
Copper	31%
Vitamin B1 (Thiamine)	28%
Iron	26%
Magnesium	19%
"Good" Fat	17%
Zinc	16%
Protein	13%
Fiber	12%
Vitamin B5 (Pantothenic Acid)	12%

12. Ginger Root

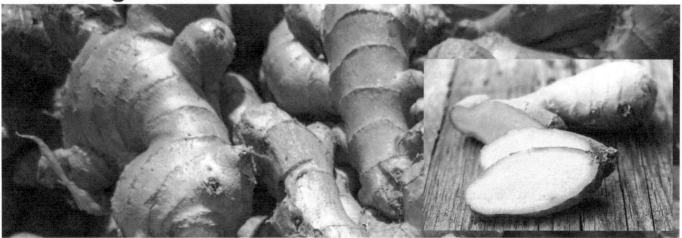

What is Ginger Root?

Ginger root, derived from the Zingiber officinale plant, is a flavorful and aromatic spice widely recognized for its culinary and medicinal properties. Rich in bioactive compounds like gingerol, ginger possesses anti-inflammatory and antioxidant effects, contributing to overall health. It is renowned for aiding digestion by alleviating nausea, indigestion, and gastrointestinal discomfort.

Additionally, ginger has potential anti-nausea benefits, making it a natural remedy for motion sickness, morning sickness during pregnancy, and chemotherapy-induced nausea. It may also help reduce muscle pain and soreness due to its anti-inflammatory properties.

Moreover, ginger has been associated with potential benefits for managing chronic conditions like osteoarthritis and may support cardiovascular health by lowering blood pressure and cholesterol levels. Whether incorporated into teas, added to dishes, or consumed in various forms, ginger root offers a flavorful and healthful addition to a balanced diet, promoting overall well-being.

Top Diseases/Conditions

Ginger Root identified as a top food for 23 of the Top 100 Diseases and Conditions. Of those, 4 Diseases and Conditions rank it as #1 (Golden Bullets), while 8 of them rank it between #2 and #10 (Silver Bullets).

4 Golden Bullets	Definition: #1 Top Food for each given condition (other than Water)
Gastroenteritis	Pneumonia
GERD / Heartburn	Vertigo

8 Silver Bullets	Definition: Top 10 food for each given condition (but not #1)
Allergies Rhinitis	Influenza
Common Cold / Virus	Inguinal Hernia
Gastritis	Streptococcal Pharyngitis
HIV	Tinnitus

Nutrients?

One serving (7g, 6 Calories) contains no nutrients that are at least 10% DRI.

13. Eggs

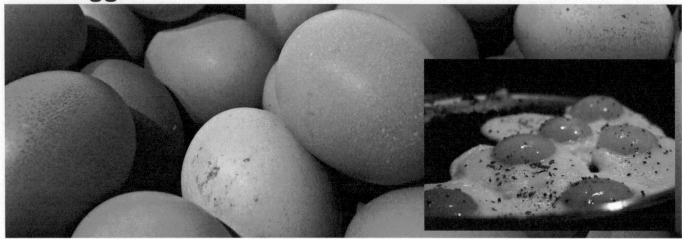

What are Eggs?

Chicken eggs, the reproductive bodies of domestic hens, are nutrient-dense and versatile food items. Rich in vitamin B7, also known as biotin, eggs contribute to energy metabolism, skin health, and the maintenance of healthy hair. Additionally, eggs are a good source of selenium, an essential mineral with antioxidant properties that support immune function and thyroid health.

Eggs also contain choline, a vital nutrient that plays a crucial role in brain development, liver function, and the formation of cell membranes. Choline is particularly important during pregnancy for fetal brain development.

Consuming eggs is considered healthy due to their high-quality protein, essential amino acids, and a diverse range of vitamins and minerals. They provide a balanced nutrient profile that supports muscle development, bone health, and overall well-being. Including eggs in a varied and balanced diet contributes to meeting nutritional needs and supporting various bodily functions.

Top Diseases/Conditions

Eggs are identified as a top food for 41 of the Top 100 Diseases and Conditions. Of those, 6 Diseases and Conditions rank it as #1 (Golden Bullets), while 14 of them rank it between #2 and #10 (Silver Bullets).

6 Golden Bullets	Definition: #1 Top Food for each given condition (other than Water)
Chronic Kidney Disease	Hyperthyroidism
Epilepsy	Obesity
Gout	Pregnancy

14 Silver Bullets	Definition: Top 10 food for each given condition (but not #1)
ADHD	Hypothyroidism
Alopecia Areata	Inflammatory Bowel Disease
Anxiety Disorder	Irritable Bowel Syndrome (IBS)
Cancer: Thyroid	Menopause
Celiac Disease	Shingles (Herpes Zoster)
Conjunctivitis	Streptococcal Pharyngitis
Gastroenteritis	Syncope

Nutrients?

One serving (Lg Egg, 55g, 80 Calories) contains:

10 Significant Nutrients	
Nutrient	DRI Per Serving (Daily Recommended Intake)
Vitamin B7 (Biotin)	33%
Selenium	32%
Vitamin B12	29%
Choline	26%
Vitamin B2 (Riboflavin)	23%
Vitamin B5 (Pantothenic Acid)	16%
Phosphorus	15%
Iron	13%
Protein	13%
Copper	11%

14. Oranges

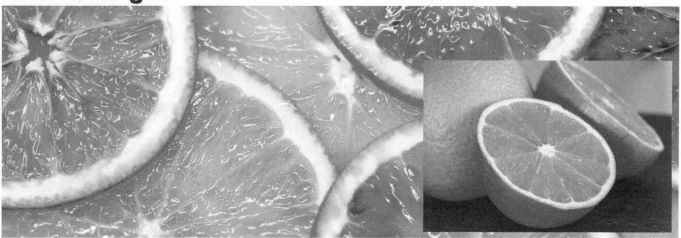

What are Oranges?

Oranges, citrus fruits from the Citrus sinensis plant, are renowned for their vibrant flavor and nutritional benefits. High in vitamin C, oranges are a powerful antioxidant that supports immune function, collagen synthesis for skin health, and acts as a cellular protector. They also contain vitamin A, primarily in the form of beta-carotene, contributing to vision health, immune support, and skin integrity.

Eating oranges is healthy due to their rich nutrient profile, including fiber, potassium, and various antioxidants. The combination of these nutrients promotes cardiovascular health, aids digestion, and may help regulate blood pressure. Oranges' natural sugars provide a quick energy boost, and their hydrating properties make them a refreshing snack.

Incorporating oranges into a balanced diet supports overall well-being, providing essential vitamins and antioxidants that contribute to immune resilience, skin health, and various physiological functions.

Top Diseases/Conditions

Oranges are identified as a top food for 42 of the Top 100 Diseases and Conditions. Of those, 10 Diseases and Conditions rank it as #1 (Golden Bullets), while 15 of them rank it between #2 and #10 (Silver Bullets).

10 Golden Bullets	Definition: #1 Top Food for each given condition (other than Water)
Arrhythmia / Afib	Gout
Congenital Heart Defect	Heart Failure
Coronary Artery Disease	HIV
Gallstones	Plantar Warts
Glaucoma	Valvular Heart Disease

15 Silver Bullets	Definition: Top 10 food for each given condition (but not #1)
Allergies Rhinitis	Conjunctivitis
Alzheimer's / Dementia	COPD
Aortic Aneurysm	Influenza
Cancer: Bladder	Multiple Sclerosis
Cancer: Colon	Peripheral Artery Disease
Cancer: Skin / Melanoma	Tuberculosis (TB)
Cataracts	Type II Diabetes
Common Cold / Virus	

Nutrients?

One serving (1 Orange, 154g, 72 Calories) contains:

6 Significant Nutrients	
Nutrient	DRI Per Serving (Daily Recommended Intake)
Vitamin C	91%
Vitamin A	39%
Vitamin B1 (Thiamine)	13%
Vitamin B6	12%
Vitamin B9 (Folate)	12%
Fiber	10%

15. Blueberries

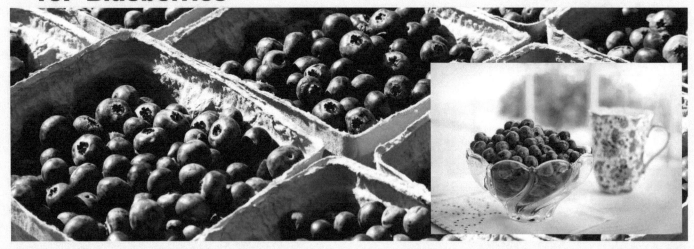

What are Blueberries?

Blueberries, small and vibrant berries from the Vaccinium genus, are celebrated for their sweet taste and numerous health benefits. Packed with antioxidants, particularly anthocyanins, blueberries have anti-inflammatory properties that contribute to overall well-being. These antioxidants help protect cells from oxidative stress and may support cardiovascular health.

Rich in vitamin K, along with dietary fiber, blueberries support immune function, collagen synthesis, and digestive health. The presence of flavonoids in blueberries is associated with cognitive benefits, potentially aiding in memory and brain function.

Furthermore, blueberries are low in calories and naturally sweet, making them a nutritious snack. Their potential role in managing oxidative stress, supporting heart health, and contributing to cognitive function makes blueberries a valuable addition to a balanced diet, promoting both deliciousness and health.

Top Diseases/Conditions

Blueberries are identified as a top food for 53 of the Top 100 Diseases and Conditions. Of those, 10

Diseases and Conditions rank it as #1 (Golden Bullets), while 22 of them rank it between #2 and #10 (Silver Bullets).

10 Golden Bullets	Definition: #1 Top Food for each given condition (other than Water)
Arrhythmia / Afib	Heart Failure
Chronic Kidney Disease	Pelvic Inflammatory Disease
Congenital Heart Defect	Peptic Ulcer
Coronary Artery Disease	Psoriasis
Epilepsy	Valvular Heart Disease

22 Silver Bullets	Definition: Top 10 food for each given condition (but not #1)
Acne	Menopause
Alzheimer's / Dementia	Obesity
Anxiety Disorder	OCD
Cancer: Bladder	Parkinson's
Cancer: Breast	Pneumonia
Cancer: Prostate	Streptococcal Pharyngitis
Chronic Liver Disease	Stroke / TIA
Depression	Tuberculosis (TB)
Gastritis	Type I Diabetes
Hemorrhoids	Type II Diabetes
Influenza	Urinary Tract Infection

Nutrients?

One serving (74g, 42 Calories) contains:

2 Significant Nutrients	
Nutrient	DRI Per Serving (Daily Recommended Intake)
Vitamin K	12%
Manganese	11%

16. Brown Rice

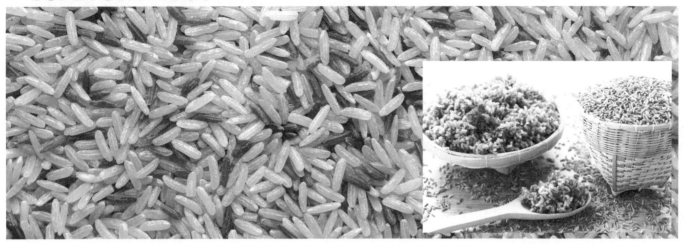

What is Brown Rice?

Brown rice, a whole grain rice variant with the bran intact, is a nutritious and gluten-free staple. Rich in manganese, brown rice supports bone development, metabolism, and antioxidant enzyme function. Manganese also contributes to collagen formation and overall connective tissue health.

Being gluten-free makes brown rice an excellent choice for those with gluten sensitivities or celiac disease, providing a safe alternative to gluten-containing grains. Additionally, brown rice contains dietary fiber, which supports digestive health, regulates blood sugar levels, and contributes to a feeling of fullness.

The health benefits of brown rice stem from its nutrient density, providing essential minerals, complex carbohydrates, and dietary fiber. As a whole grain, it retains more nutrients compared to refined grains. Incorporating brown rice into a balanced diet promotes overall well-being, offering sustained energy, supporting digestive health, and contributing to a nutrient-rich and gluten-free dietary choice.

Top Diseases/Conditions

Brown Rice is identified as a top food for 39 of the Top 100 Diseases and Conditions. Of those, 4 Diseases and Conditions rank it as #1 (Golden Bullets), while 14 of them rank it between #2 and #10 (Silver Bullets).

4 Golden Bullets	Definition: #1 Top Food for each given condition (other than Water)
Gastroenteritis	Kidney Stone
GERD / Heartburn	Rheumatoid Arthritis

14 Silver Bullets	Definition: Top 10 food for each given condition (but not #1)
Aortic Aneurysm	HIV
Brain Tumors	Inguinal Hernia
Cancer: Breast	Insomnia
Cancer: Colon	Parkinson's
Diverticulitis	Stroke / TIA
Fibromyalgia	Syncope
Hemorrhoids	Tuberculosis (TB)

Nutrients?

One serving (1/6 Cup Uncooked, 46g, 171 Calories) or (1/2 Cup Cooked, 131g, 171 Calories) contains:

9 Significant Nutrients	
Nutrient	DRI Per Serving (Daily Recommended Intake)
Manganese	75%
Phosphorus	22%
Selenium	20%
Vitamin B6	17%
Magnesium	16%
Vitamin B3 (Niacin)	15%
Vitamin B1 (Thiamine)	15%
Vitamin B5 (Pantothenic Acid)	14%
Copper	14%

17. Walnuts

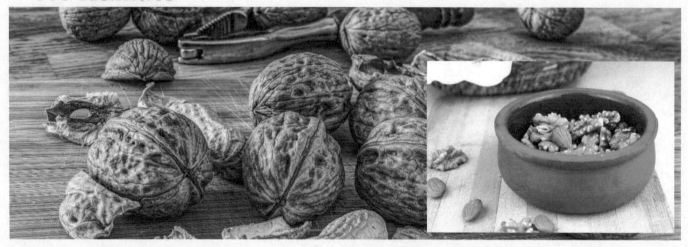

What are Walnuts?

Walnuts, the seeds of the Juglans regia tree, are nutrient-dense nuts known for their distinctive flavor and numerous health benefits. Rich in omega-3 alpha-linolenic acid (ALA) and omega-6 fatty acids, walnuts contribute to heart health, brain function, and inflammation regulation. The balance between omega-3 ALA and omega-6 fatty acids in walnuts supports a healthy ratio, which is crucial for overall well-being.

In addition to healthy fats, walnuts contain antioxidants, vitamins, and minerals, including copper and manganese. These compounds contribute to cellular protection and bone health.

Consuming walnuts is associated with various health benefits, such as improving heart health, reducing inflammation, and supporting brain function. Incorporating walnuts into a balanced diet provides a tasty and nutritious way to obtain essential nutrients, promoting overall health and well-being.

Top Diseases/Conditions

Walnuts are identified as a top food for 58 of the Top 100 Diseases and Conditions. Of those, 11 Diseases and Conditions rank it as #1 (Golden Bullets), while 28 of them rank it between #2 and #10 (Silver Bullets).

11 Golden Bullets	Definition: #1 Top Food for each given condition (other than Water)
Arrhythmia / Afib	Heart Failure
Cancer: Uterus / Endometrial	Osteoarthritis
Cardiomyopathy	Peripheral Artery Disease
Congenital Heart Defect	Type II Diabetes
Coronary Artery Disease	Valvular Heart Disease
Gout	

28 Silver Bullets	Definition: Top 10 food for each given condition (but not #1)
Allergies Rhinitis	Hepatitis B
Alopecia Areata	Hepatitis C
Anxiety Disorder	High Cholesterol
Atopic Dermatitis	Insomnia
Cancer: Bladder	Lumbar Radiculopathy
Cancer: Non-Hodgkin's Lymphoma	Multiple Sclerosis
Celiac Disease	Parkinson's
Chlamydia	Pelvic Inflammatory Disease
Contact Dermatitis	Psoriasis
Depression	Raynaud's Syndrome
Endometriosis	Rheumatoid Arthritis
Fibromyalgia	Rosacea
Gallstones	Sleep Apnea
GERD / Heartburn	Tinnitus

Nutrients?

One serving (28g, 183 Calories) contains:

9 Significant Nutrients	
Nutrient	DRI Per Serving (Daily Recommended Intake)
Omega-3 ALA	159%
Omega 6 LA	63%
Copper	44%
Manganese	43%
"Good" Fat	36%
Vitamin B6	15%
Phosphorus	14%
Magnesium	11%
Iron	10%

18. Greek Yogurt

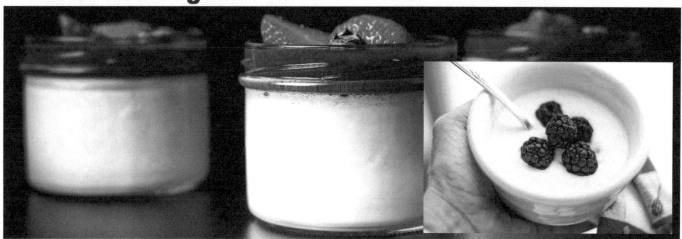

What is Greek Yogurt?

Greek yogurt is a thick and creamy yogurt variant that undergoes straining to remove excess whey, resulting in a higher protein content. Rich in vitamin B12, Greek yogurt supports energy metabolism, neurological function, and the formation of red blood cells. Additionally, it is an excellent source of calcium, essential for bone health, muscle function, and blood clotting.

Greek yogurt contains probiotics, beneficial bacteria that promote gut health and support the digestive system. These probiotics contribute to a balanced gut microbiome, potentially enhancing immune function and nutrient absorption.

The health benefits of Greek yogurt extend to its protein content, aiding in muscle repair and satiety. Its nutrient profile, including vitamins, minerals, and probiotics, makes Greek yogurt a nutritious option for a well-rounded diet. Incorporating Greek yogurt into meals and snacks provides a delicious and healthful way to support overall well-being.

Top Diseases/Conditions

Greek Yogurt is identified as a top food for 45 of the Top 100 Diseases and Conditions. Of those, 8 Diseases and Conditions rank it as #1 (Golden Bullets), while 16 of them rank it between #2 and #10 (Silver Bullets).

8 Golden Bullets	Definition: #1 Top Food for each given condition (other than Water)
Gastritis	Premenstrual Syndrome
Lumbar Radiculopathy	Type I Diabetes
Oral / Dental Health	Type II Diabetes
Peptic Ulcer	Urinary Tract Infection

16 Silver Bullets	Definition: Top 10 food for each given condition (but not #1)
Anxiety Disorder	HIV
Cancer: Thyroid	Hyperthyroidism
Chlamydia	Hypothyroidism
Cold Sores	Inflammatory Bowel Disease
Constipation	Obesity
Depression	Osteoporosis
Fibromyalgia	Pregnancy
Genital Herpes	Streptococcal Pharyngitis

Nutrients?

One serving (245g, 154 Calories) contains:

11 Significant Nutrients	
Nutrient	DRI Per Serving (Daily Recommended Intake)
Vitamin B12	58%
Phosphorus	50%
Calcium	45%
Vitamin B2 (Riboflavin)	38%
Vitamin B5 (Pantothenic Acid)	28%
Protein	23%
Zinc	20%
Potassium	17%
Selenium	15%
Sodium	11%
Magnesium	10%

19. Garlic Cloves

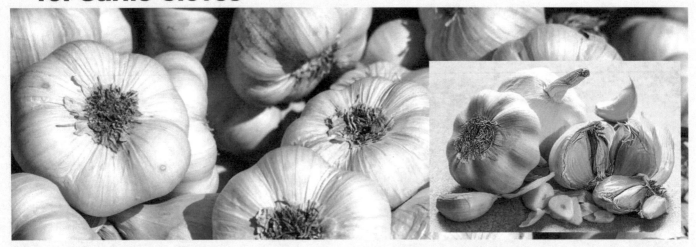

What are Garlic Cloves?

Garlic, Allium sativum, is a flavorful and aromatic bulb commonly used as both a culinary ingredient and a traditional medicinal remedy. Rich in bioactive compounds, particularly allicin, garlic exhibits various health benefits. Allicin is known for its antimicrobial properties, potentially supporting the immune system and combating infections.

Garlic is associated with cardiovascular benefits, such as lowering blood pressure and cholesterol levels, reducing the risk of heart disease. Its anti-inflammatory and antioxidant properties may contribute to overall cardiovascular health. Additionally, garlic is recognized for its potential in supporting immune function, promoting detoxification, and offering anti-cancer properties.

Incorporating garlic into a balanced diet, whether raw or cooked, adds depth of flavor and a range of health-promoting compounds, making it a valuable and tasty addition to various culinary creations with potential positive impacts on overall well-being.

Top Diseases/Conditions

Garlic Cloves are identified as a top food for 33 of the Top 100 Diseases and Conditions. Of those, 3 Diseases and Conditions rank it as #1 (Golden Bullets), while 13 of them rank it between #2 and #10 (Silver Bullets).

3 Golden Bullets	Definition: #1 Top Food for each given condition (other than Water)
Chlamydia	Common Cold / Virus
Chronic Liver Disease	

13 Silver Bullets	Definition: Top 10 food for each given condition (but not #1)
Allergies Rhinitis	Multiple Sclerosis
Brain Tumors	Oral / Dental Health
Cancer: Bladder	Plantar Warts
Cancer: Colon	Pneumonia
Chronic Kidney Disease	Raynaud's Syndrome
Hepatitis C	Syncope
Hepatitis B	Urinary Tract Infection

Nutrients?

One serving (3g, 5 Calories) contains no nutrients that are at least 10% DRI.

20. Carrots

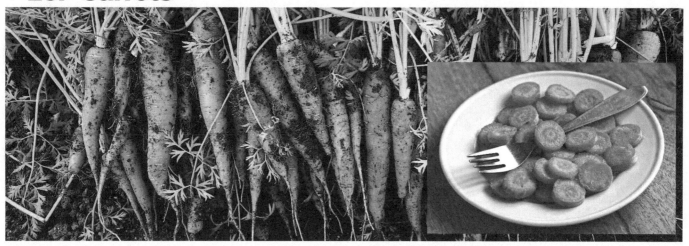

What are Carrots?

Carrots, Daucus carota, are vibrant orange root vegetables prized for their sweet taste and nutritional richness. They are a robust source of beta-carotene, a precursor to vitamin A, which plays a pivotal role in maintaining healthy vision, supporting the immune system, and promoting skin integrity. The high beta-carotene content gives carrots their distinctive color and serves as a potent antioxidant, protecting cells from oxidative stress.

Eating carrots is healthy due to their nutrient density, offering a range of vitamins, minerals, and fiber. They contribute to overall well-being by promoting digestive health, supporting a strong immune system, and providing essential nutrients for skin and eye health. Incorporating carrots into a balanced diet adds a delicious and nutritious element, contributing to various aspects of health and vitality.

Top Diseases/Conditions

Carrots are identified as a top food for 39 of the Top 100 Diseases and Conditions. Of those, 4 Diseases and Conditions rank it as #1 (Golden Bullets), while 17 of them rank it between #2 and #10 (Silver Bullets).

4 Golden Bullets	Definition: #1 Top Food for each given condition (other than Water)
Cancer: Breast	Kidney Stone
Cataracts	Tuberculosis (TB)

17 Silver Bullets	Definition: Top 10 food for each given condition (but not #1)
Acne	Glaucoma
Asthma	Hepatitis B
Brain Tumors	HIV
Cancer: Skin / Melanoma	Irritable Bowel Syndrome (IBS)
Conjunctivitis	Migrain
COPD	Oral / Dental Health
Diverticulitis	Plantar Warts
Fibroids	Shingles (Herpes Zoster)
GERD / Heartburn	

Nutrients?

One serving (78g, 32 Calories) contains:

1 Significant Nutrient	
Nutrient	DRI Per Serving (Daily Recommended Intake)
Vitamin A	434%

21. Avocados

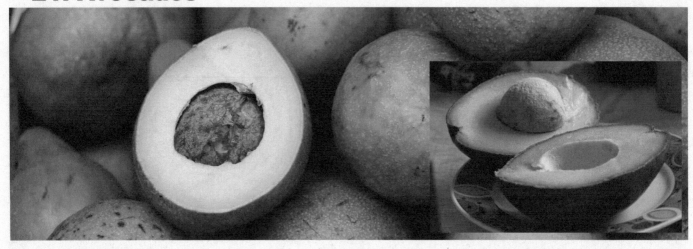

What are Avocados?

Avocados, fruits from the Persea americana tree, are nutritional powerhouses rich in monounsaturated fats, particularly oleic acid, which supports heart health by reducing bad cholesterol levels and promoting good cholesterol. They also contain vitamin B5 (pantothenic acid), contributing to energy metabolism, hormone synthesis, and overall cellular function. Additionally, avocados provide folate, essential for DNA synthesis and cell division, making them particularly beneficial during pregnancy.

The combination of monounsaturated fats, vitamins, and minerals in avocados offers a range of health benefits. These include supporting cardiovascular health, promoting healthy skin, aiding in energy production, and contributing to the development of a healthy nervous system. Incorporating avocados into a balanced diet adds a delicious and nutrient-dense food that supports overall well-being, showcasing the diverse range of health-promoting compounds found in this versatile fruit.

Top Diseases/Conditions

Avocados are identified as a top food for 41 of the Top 100 Diseases and Conditions. Of those, 5 Diseases and Conditions rank it as #1 (Golden Bullets), while 9 of them rank it between #2 and #10 (Silver Bullets).

5 Golden Bullets	Definition: #1 Top Food for each given condition (other than Water)
Chronic Liver Disease	Kidney Stone
Depression	Obesity
Gout	

9 Silver Bullets	Definition: Top 10 food for each given condition (but not #1)
Celiac Disease	HIV
Diverticulitis	Plantar Warts
Epilepsy	Pneumonia
Hepatitis B	Tinnitus
High Cholesterol	

Nutrients?

One serving (50g, 80 Calories) contains:

5 Significant Nutrients	
Nutrient	DRI Per Serving (Daily Recommended Intake)
Vitamin B5 (Pantothenic Acid)	14%
"Good" Fat	13%
Copper	11%
Vitamin B9 (Folate)	10%
Vitamin B6	10%

22. Bananas

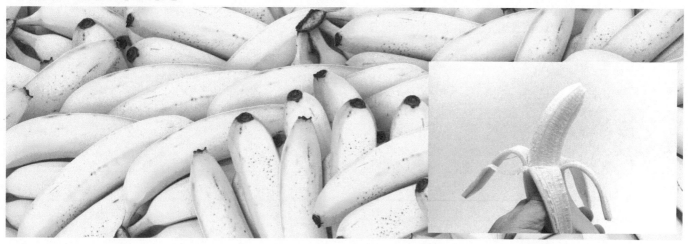

What are Bananas?

Bananas, fruits from the Musa species, are not only a convenient and delicious snack but also offer notable health benefits. Rich in vitamin B6, bananas play a crucial role in cognitive development, immune function, and the synthesis of neurotransmitters. They are an excellent source of potassium, essential for maintaining proper blood pressure, fluid balance, and supporting heart health. Additionally, bananas contain manganese, contributing to bone health, metabolism, and antioxidant defense.

The healthiness of bananas stems from their nutrient-rich profile, providing a quick and natural energy boost from natural sugars and a variety of essential vitamins and minerals. Their dietary fiber content supports digestive health, and the combination of nutrients makes bananas a nutritious and convenient option for supporting overall well-being, making them a popular and versatile fruit in a balanced diet.

Top Diseases/Conditions

Bananas are identified as a top food for 29 of the Top 100 Diseases and Conditions. Of those, 5 Diseases and Conditions rank it as #1 (Golden Bullets), while 2 of them rank it between #2 and #10 (Silver Bullets).

5 Golden Bullets	Definition: #1 Top Food for each given condition (other than Water)
Aortic Aneurysm	Kidney Stone
Gastroenteritis	Tinnitus
Hypertension	

2 Silver Bullets	Definition: Top 10 food for each given condition (but not #1)
Autism	Syncope

Nutrients?

One serving (126g, 112 Calories) contains:

5 Significant Nutrients	
Nutrient	DRI Per Serving (Daily Recommended Intake)
Vitamin B6	38%
Potassium	13%
Manganese	13%
Vitamin C	12%
Copper	11%

23. Lemons

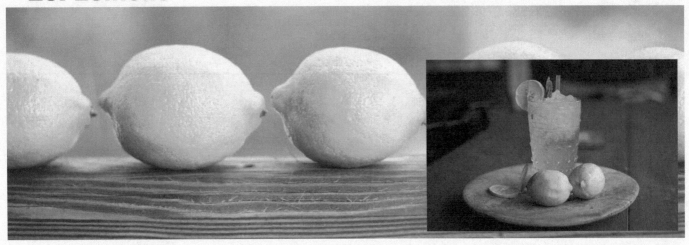

What are Lemons?

Lemons, citrus fruits from the Citrus limon tree, are celebrated for their tangy flavor and various health benefits. Rich in vitamin C, lemons support immune function, skin health, and act as a powerful antioxidant, protecting cells from oxidative stress. They also contain flavonoids, compounds with anti-inflammatory and potential anti-cancer properties.

The acidity of lemons aids in digestion and may enhance the absorption of certain nutrients. Furthermore, lemons contribute to hydration and may assist in weight management by promoting a feeling of fullness.

Incorporating lemons into a balanced diet adds a burst of refreshing flavor and essential nutrients. Whether squeezed over salads, used in beverages, or as a zesty addition to recipes, lemons offer a delicious and healthful way to enhance both the taste and nutritional value of meals, supporting overall well-being.

Top Diseases/Conditions

Lemons are identified as a top food for 25 of the Top 100 Diseases and Conditions. Of those, 4 Diseases and Conditions rank it as #1 (Golden Bullets), while 6 of them rank it between #2 and #10 (Silver Bullets).

4 Golden Bullets	Definition: #1 Top Food for each given condition (other than Water)
Chronic Liver Disease	Gallstones
Common Cold / Virus	Influenza

6 Silver Bullets	Definition: Top 10 food for each given condition (but not #1)
Allergies Rhinitis	Cancer: Skin / Melanoma
Aortic Aneurysm	Glaucoma
Cancer: Colon	Hepatitis B

Nutrients?

One serving (58g, 17 Calories) contains:

1 Significant Nutrient	
Nutrient	DRI Per Serving (Daily Recommended Intake)
Vitamin C	34%

24. Herring

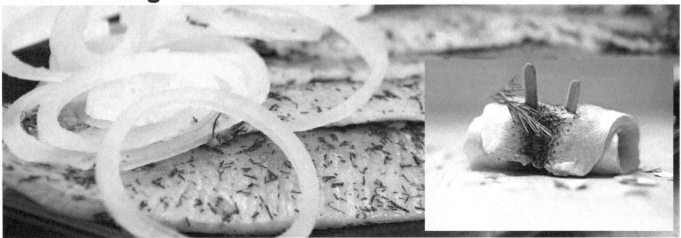

What is Herring?

Herrings, oily fish belonging to the Clupeidae family, are nutritional powerhouses with numerous health benefits. Rich in vitamin B12, herrings contribute to nerve function, DNA synthesis, and red blood cell formation. They are also abundant in omega-3 fatty acids, specifically DHA (docosahexaenoic acid) and EPA (eicosapentaenoic acid), supporting heart health, cognitive function, and reducing inflammation.

Herrings are an excellent source of vitamin D, essential for calcium absorption, bone health, and immune system support. The combination of omega-3s and vitamin D makes herrings particularly valuable for overall well-being.

Regular consumption of herrings is associated with cardiovascular benefits, improved brain health, and reduced inflammation. Their nutrient profile, including essential vitamins and omega-3 fatty acids, makes herrings a delicious and healthful addition to a balanced diet, offering a diverse range of benefits for various aspects of health.

Top Diseases/Conditions

Herring is identified as a top food for 60 of the Top 100 Diseases and Conditions. Of those, 14 Diseases and Conditions rank it as #1 (Golden Bullets), while 23 of them rank it between #2 and #10 (Silver Bullets).

14 Golden Bullets	Definition: #1 Top Food for each given condition (other than Water)
Arrhythmia / Afib	Heart Failure
Autism	Multiple Sclerosis
Cancer: Skin / Melanoma	Parkinson's
Cancer: Uterus / Endometrial	Pelvic Inflammatory Disease
Cardiomyopathy	Psoriasis
Congenital Heart Defect	Schizophrenia
Coronary Artery Disease	Valvular Heart Disease

23 Silver Bullets	Definition: Top 10 food for each given condition (but not #1)
ADHD	Hepatitis C
Alzheimer's / Dementia	Inflammatory Bowel Disease
Atopic Dermatitis	Insomnia
Bipolar Disorder	Irritable Bowel Syndrome (IBS)
Cancer: Colon	Migrain
Cancer: Non-Hodgkin's Lymphoma	Mononucleosis
Cancer: Prostate	Pneumonia
Cold Sores	Rheumatoid Arthritis
Contact Dermatitis	Stroke / TIA
Depression	Tuberculosis (TB)
Endometriosis	Type I Diabetes
Glaucoma	

Nutrients?

One serving (85g, 134 Calories) contains:

15 Significant Nutrients	
Nutrient	DRI Per Serving (Daily Recommended Intake)
Vitamin B12	483%
Omega-3 DHA	293%
Omega-3 EPA	241%
Vitamin D	231%
Selenium	56%
Phosphorus	29%
Protein	27%
Vitamin B6	23%
Vitamin B3 (Niacin)	17%
Vitamin B2 (Riboflavin)	15%
"Good" Fat	11%
Iron	11%
Copper	11%
Choline	10%
Vitamin B5 (Pantothenic Acid)	10%

25. Extra Virgin Olive Oil

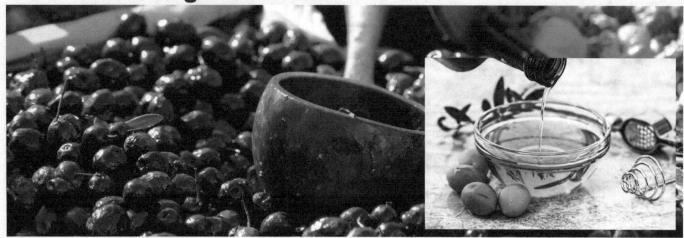

What is Extra Virgin Olive Oil?

Extra virgin olive oil (EVOO) is a premium quality oil extracted from olives, known for its rich flavor and health-promoting properties. Primarily composed of monounsaturated fats, EVOO contains oleic acid, which supports heart health by reducing bad cholesterol levels and improving overall lipid profiles. It is also a good source of vitamin E, a potent antioxidant that protects cells from oxidative stress, supports skin health, and contributes to immune function.

The monounsaturated fats in EVOO provide a healthy option for cooking and dressing, promoting satiety and aiding in weight management. The presence of polyphenols, another group of antioxidants in EVOO, further contributes to its anti-inflammatory and cardiovascular benefits.

Incorporating extra virgin olive oil into a balanced diet offers a delicious way to enhance flavors while reaping the numerous health benefits associated with its nutrient-rich profile and heart-healthy fats.

Top Diseases/Conditions

Extra Virgin Olive Oil is identified as a top food for 42 of the Top 100 Diseases and Conditions. Of those, 4 Diseases and Conditions rank it as #1 (Golden Bullets), while 5 of them rank it between #2 and #10 (Silver Bullets).

4 Golden Bullets	Definition: #1 Top Food for each given condition (other than Water)
Chronic Liver Disease	Pelvic Inflammatory Disease
Hepatitis B	Rheumatoid Arthritis

5 Silver Bullets	Definition: Top 10 food for each given condition (but not #1)
Cardiomyopathy	Type I Diabetes
High Cholesterol	Vertigo
Osteoarthritis	

Nutrients?

One serving (13g, 119 Calories) contains:

2 Significant Nutrients	
Nutrient	DRI Per Serving (Daily Recommended Intake)
"Good" Fat	25%
Vitamin E	13%

26. Sweet Potatoes

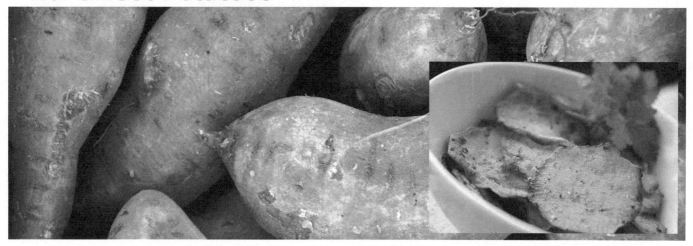

What are Sweet Potatoes?

Sweet potatoes, the root vegetables from the Ipomoea batatas plant, are not only a tasty addition to meals but also offer impressive health benefits. Rich in beta-carotene, sweet potatoes are a potent source of vitamin A, supporting vision, immune function, and skin health. The high fiber content aids digestion, promoting a healthy gut and contributing to satiety, which may assist in weight management.

Sweet potatoes also provide essential vitamins like vitamin C, B vitamins, and minerals such as potassium and manganese. The combination of nutrients and antioxidants in sweet potatoes contributes to overall well-being, including anti-inflammatory and anti-cancer properties.

Their natural sweetness makes sweet potatoes a versatile and nutritious choice for various culinary applications. Incorporating them into a balanced diet not only adds flavor and texture but also provides a range of essential nutrients, supporting multiple aspects of health.

Top Diseases/Conditions

Sweet Potatoes are identified as a top food for 36 of the Top 100 Diseases and Conditions. Of those, 1 Diseases and Conditions rank it as #1 (Golden Bullets), while 12 of them rank it between #2 and #10 (Silver Bullets).

1 Golden Bullet	Definition: #1 Top Food for each given condition (other than Water)
Cancer: Bladder	

12 Silver Bullets	Definition: Top 10 food for each given condition (but not #1)
Asthma	Glaucoma
Brain Tumors	Irritable Bowel Syndrome (IBS)
Conjunctivitis	Migrain
Diverticulitis	Pregnancy
Fibroids	Sleep Apnea
GERD / Heartburn	Tuberculosis (TB)

Nutrients?

One serving (130g, 112 Calories) contains:

8 Significant Nutrients	
Nutrient	DRI Per Serving (Daily Recommended Intake)
Vitamin A	615%
Vitamin B6	23%
Copper	22%
Vitamin B5 (Pantothenic Acid)	20%
Manganese	13%
Potassium	13%
Fiber	10%
Iron	10%

27. Tomatoes

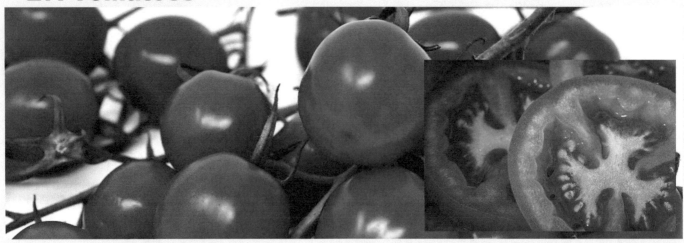

What are Tomatoes?

Tomatoes, the vibrant fruits of the Solanum lycopersicum plant, are not only a culinary staple but also offer a wealth of health benefits. Packed with nutrients, tomatoes are a rich source of vitamin A, supporting vision, immune function, and skin health. Additionally, they contain antioxidants like lycopene, known for its potential to reduce the risk of certain cancers and support heart health.

Tomatoes are low in calories and high in essential vitamins such as vitamin C, potassium, and copper. Their high water content contributes to hydration, and the presence of dietary fiber promotes digestive health.

Incorporating tomatoes into a balanced diet adds a burst of flavor, essential nutrients, and antioxidants. Whether eaten fresh, cooked in dishes, or enjoyed in sauces, tomatoes provide a delicious and healthful addition to meals, supporting overall well-being.

Top Diseases/Conditions

Tomatoes are identified as a top food for 36 of the Top 100 Diseases and Conditions. Of those, 3 Diseases and Conditions rank it as #1 (Golden Bullets), while 8 of them rank it between #2 and #10 (Silver Bullets).

3 Golden Bullets	Definition: #1 Top Food for each given condition (other than Water)
Brain Tumors	Tuberculosis (TB)
Cancer: Prostate	

8 Silver Bullets	Definition: Top 10 food for each given condition (but not #1)
Anemia of Chronic Disease	Iron Deficiency Anemia
Cancer: Colon	Mononucleosis
Cataracts	Sleep Apnea
Conjunctivitis	Type I Diabetes

Nutrients?

One serving (148g, 27 Calories) contains:

5 Significant Nutrients	
Nutrient	DRI Per Serving (Daily Recommended Intake)
Vitamin A	41%
Vitamin C	21%
Copper	11%
Potassium	10%
Vitamin K	10%

28. Sardines

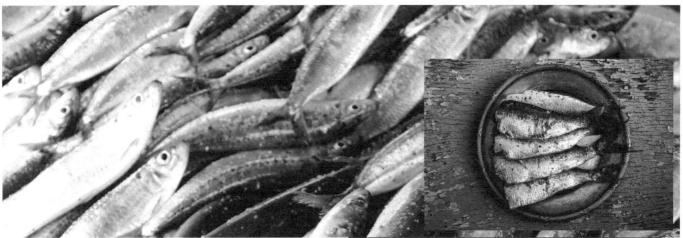

What are Sardines?

Sardines, small oily fish belonging to the herring family, are nutritional powerhouses with numerous health benefits. Rich in vitamin B12, sardines support nerve function, red blood cell production, and overall energy metabolism. They are also abundant in omega-3 fatty acids, particularly DHA (docosahexaenoic acid) and EPA (eicosapentaenoic acid), essential for heart health, cognitive function, and reducing inflammation.

Sardines are an excellent source of selenium, a vital mineral with antioxidant properties that support immune function and protect against oxidative stress. The combination of omega-3s and selenium in sardines contributes to overall cardiovascular well-being and may reduce the risk of chronic diseases.

Incorporating sardines into a balanced diet provides a convenient and nutrient-dense source of essential vitamins, minerals, and omega-3 fatty acids, supporting various aspects of health, making them a valuable addition to a health-conscious eating plan.

Top Diseases/Conditions

Sardines are identified as a top food for 38 of the Top 100 Diseases and Conditions. Of those, 3 Diseases and Conditions rank it as #1 (Golden Bullets), while 10 of them rank it between #2 and #10 (Silver Bullets).

3 Golden Bullets	Definition: #1 Top Food for each given condition (other than Water)
Alopecia Areata	Premenstrual Syndrome
Atopic Dermatitis	

10 Silver Bullets	Definition: Top 10 food for each given condition (but not #1)
Anemia of Chronic Disease	Menopause
Cold Sores	Migrain
Hyperthyroidism	Osteoporosis
Hypothyroidism	Pelvic Inflammatory Disease
Irritable Bowel Syndrome (IBS)	Shingles (Herpes Zoster)

Nutrients?

One serving (85g, 177 Calories) contains:

21 Significant Nutrients	
Nutrient	DRI Per Serving (Daily Recommended Intake)
Vitamin B12	316%
Omega-3 DHA	173%
Omega-3 EPA	161%
Selenium	81%
Phosphorus	59%
Vitamin D	39%
Protein	37%
Calcium	32%
Iron	31%
Sodium	29%
Vitamin B3 (Niacin)	28%
Omega-3 ALA	26%
Copper	19%
Omega 6 LA	18%
"Good" Fat	18%
Choline	13%
Vitamin B2 (Riboflavin)	13%
Vitamin E	11%
Vitamin B5 (Pantothenic Acid)	11%
Zinc	10%
Potassium	10%

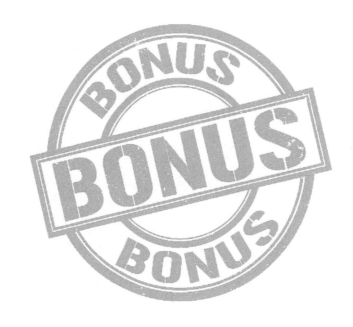

Top 10 Most Nutrient Dense Foods in the Top 100	
Food	**# of Nutrients**
Sardines	21
Soybeans	20
Peas	17
Beef Liver	17
Mackeral	16
Sunflower Seeds	15
Salmon	14
Herring	14
Oysters	14
Broccoli	13
Peanuts	13

29. Grapefruit

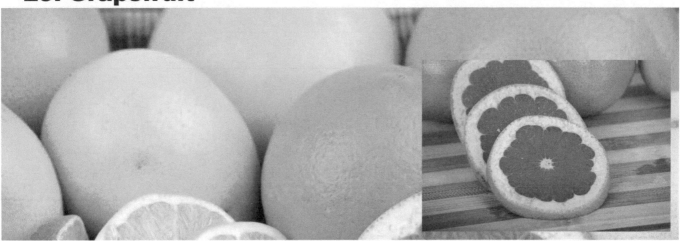

What is Grapefruit?

Grapefruits, citrus fruits from the Citrus paradisi tree, offer a refreshing burst of flavor along with notable health benefits. Rich in vitamin C, grapefruits contribute to a robust immune system, collagen synthesis, and antioxidant defense, promoting skin health and overall well-being. They also contain vitamin A, important for vision, immune function, and skin health.

The combination of vitamins, fiber, and antioxidants in grapefruits makes them a nutritious choice for supporting cardiovascular health, managing weight, and reducing the risk of chronic diseases. The presence of bioactive compounds, such as flavonoids and carotenoids, contributes to their anti-inflammatory and potential anti-cancer properties.

Incorporating grapefruits into a balanced diet provides a delicious way to boost vitamin intake and enjoy the numerous health benefits associated with their nutrient-rich profile, making them a flavorful and healthful addition to meals and snacks.

Top Diseases/Conditions

Grapefruit is identified as a top food for 29 of the Top 100 Diseases and Conditions. Of those, 2 Diseases and Conditions rank it as #1 (Golden Bullets), while 6 of them rank it between #2 and #10 (Silver Bullets).

2 Golden Bullets	Definition: #1 Top Food for each given condition (other than Water)
Chronic Liver Disease	Gallstones

6 Silver Bullets	Definition: Top 10 food for each given condition (but not #1)
Aortic Aneurysm	COPD
Cataracts	Glaucoma
Conjunctivitis	Obesity

Nutrients?

One serving (154g, 65 Calories) contains:

2 Significant Nutrients	
Nutrient	DRI Per Serving (Daily Recommended Intake)
Vitamin A	59%
Vitamin C	53%

30. Black Beans

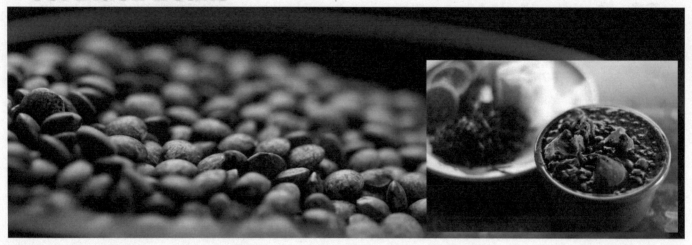

What are Black Beans?

Black beans, legumes from the Phaseolus vulgaris plant, are not only a versatile and flavorful addition to meals but also offer impressive health benefits. Rich in iron, black beans contribute to the formation of red blood cells and oxygen transport in the body, supporting energy metabolism. They also provide copper, an essential mineral involved in various physiological processes, including iron metabolism and the formation of connective tissues.

The combination of fiber, protein, and various vitamins and minerals in black beans supports digestive health, helps regulate blood sugar levels, and promotes overall well-being. Their low glycemic index makes them a suitable option for those managing blood sugar.

Incorporating black beans into a balanced diet provides a nutrient-dense source of plant-based protein, fiber, and essential minerals, offering numerous health benefits and making them a valuable component of a health-conscious eating plan.

Top Diseases/Conditions

Black Beans are identified as a top food for 46 of the Top 100 Diseases and Conditions. Of those, 5 Diseases and Conditions rank it as #1 (Golden Bullets), while 7 of them rank it between #2 and #10 (Silver Bullets).

5 Golden Bullets	Definition: #1 Top Food for each given condition (other than Water)
Arrhythmia / Afib	Heart Failure
Congenital Heart Defect	Valvular Heart Disease
Coronary Artery Disease	

7 Silver Bullets	Definition: Top 10 food for each given condition (but not #1)
ADHD	Inflammatory Bowel Disease
Chlamydia	Iron Deficiency Anemia
Gastritis	Obesity
Hemorrhoids	

Nutrients?

One serving (97g, 126 Calories) contains:

10 Significant Nutrients	
Nutrient	DRI Per Serving (Daily Recommended Intake)
Iron	35%
Copper	29%
Phosphorus	21%
Vitamin B9 (Folate)	21%
Vitamin B1 (Thiamine)	17%
Protein	14%
Manganese	14%
Fiber	14%
Potassium	12%
Magnesium	11%

31. Raspberries

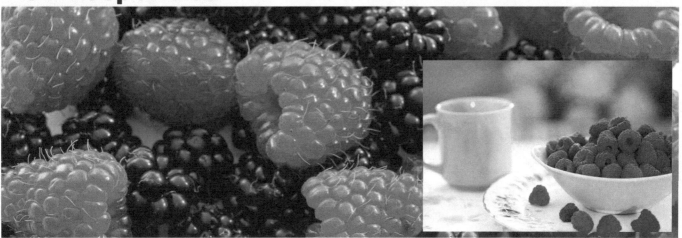

What are Raspberries?

Raspberries, vibrant berries from the Rubus idaeus plant, are not only delicious but also packed with nutritional benefits. Rich in vitamin C, raspberries support immune function, collagen synthesis, and antioxidant defense, contributing to skin health and overall well-being. They also provide manganese, a trace mineral essential for bone formation, metabolism, and antioxidant enzyme activity.

The combination of dietary fiber, vitamins, minerals, and antioxidants in raspberries makes them a healthful choice for various aspects of well-being. Their high fiber content supports digestive health, while the antioxidants, including flavonoids and polyphenols, offer potential anti-inflammatory and anti-cancer properties.

Incorporating raspberries into a balanced diet adds a burst of flavor, essential nutrients, and a range of health benefits. Whether enjoyed fresh, in smoothies, or as a topping for yogurt, raspberries are a nutritious and tasty addition to a health-conscious eating plan.

Top Diseases/Conditions

Raspberries are identified as a top food for 34 of the Top 100 Diseases and Conditions. Of those, 4 Diseases and Conditions rank it as #1 (Golden Bullets), while 1 of them rank it between #2 and #10 (Silver Bullets).

4 Golden Bullets	Definition: #1 Top Food for each given condition (other than Water)
Cancer: Uterus / Endometrial	Hemorrhoids
Epilepsy	Hypertension

1 Silver Bullet	Definition: Top 10 food for each given condition (but not #1)
Brain Tumors	Constipation

Nutrients?

One serving (125g, 65 Calories) contains:

6 Significant Nutrients	
Nutrient	DRI Per Serving (Daily Recommended Intake)
Manganese	37%
Vitamin C	36%
Fiber	21%
Copper	13%
Iron	11%
Omega-3 ALA	10%

32. Flaxseed

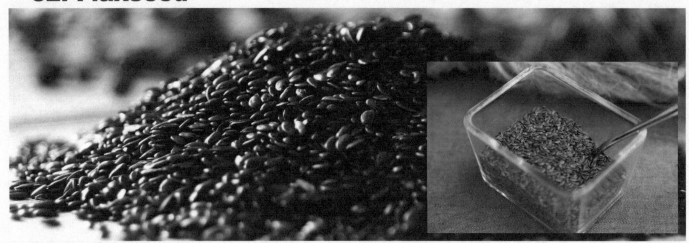

What are Flaxseeds?

Flaxseeds, tiny seeds from the Linum usitatissimum plant, are nutritional powerhouses renowned for their health benefits. Packed with omega-3 alpha-linolenic acid (ALA), flaxseeds offer a plant-based source of this essential fatty acid crucial for heart health, reducing inflammation, and supporting brain function. ALA is a precursor to other omega-3 fatty acids like EPA and DHA.

Flaxseeds are also rich in dietary fiber, which aids in digestion, promotes a feeling of fullness, and helps regulate blood sugar levels. Additionally, they contain lignans, plant compounds with antioxidant properties that may have anti-cancer effects.

Incorporating flaxseeds into a balanced diet adds a nutritional boost, providing essential fatty acids, fiber, and antioxidants. Whether ground and sprinkled on yogurt or added to smoothies, flaxseeds offer a convenient and versatile way to enhance the nutrient profile of meals, supporting overall well-being.

Top Diseases/Conditions

Flaxseeds are identified as a top food for 51 of the Top 100 Diseases and Conditions. Of those, 3 Diseases and Conditions rank it as #1 (Golden Bullets), while 12 of them rank it between #2 and #10 (Silver Bullets).

3 Golden Bullets	Definition: #1 Top Food for each given condition (other than Water)
Constipation	Pelvic Inflammatory Disease
Gallstones	

12 Silver Bullets	Definition: Top 10 food for each given condition (but not #1)
ADHD	Depression
Asthma	Lumbar Radiculopathy
Atopic Dermatitis	Menopause
Cardiomyopathy	Psoriasis
Chlamydia	Raynaud's Syndrome
Contact Dermatitis	Rosacea

Nutrients?

One serving (10g, 55 Calories) contains:

5 Significant Nutrients	
Nutrient	DRI Per Serving (Daily Recommended Intake)
Omega-3 ALA	146%
Vitamin B1 (Thiamine)	17%
Manganese	13%
Copper	11%
Magnesium	10%

33. Chia Seeds

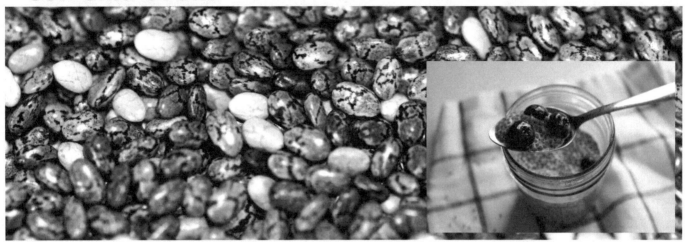

What are Chia Seeds?

Chia seeds, derived from the Salvia hispanica plant, are tiny but nutrient-dense, making them a valuable addition to a healthy diet. These seeds are particularly notable for their omega-3 fatty acid content, specifically alpha-linolenic acid (ALA). Omega-3s play a crucial role in heart health, reducing inflammation, and supporting brain function.

Chia seeds also contain omega-6 fatty acids, contributing to a balanced ratio with omega-3s. The combination of these essential fatty acids supports overall cardiovascular health and immune function. Additionally, chia seeds are rich in dietary fiber, promoting digestive health, aiding in weight management, and providing a sustained release of energy.

Incorporating chia seeds into meals, such as adding them to smoothies or yogurt, offers a convenient and versatile way to enhance nutrient intake, providing a range of essential nutrients that contribute to overall well-being.

Top Diseases/Conditions

Chia Seeds are identified as a top food for 38 of the Top 100 Diseases and Conditions. Of those, 1 Diseases and Conditions rank it as #1 (Golden Bullets), while 7 of them rank it between #2 and #10 (Silver Bullets).

1 Golden Bullet	Definition: #1 Top Food for each given condition (other than Water)
Rosacea	

7 Silver Bullets	Definition: Top 10 food for each given condition (but not #1)
Anxiety Disorder	Endometriosis
Chlamydia	Menopause
Constipation	Raynaud's Syndrome
Depression	

Nutrients?

One serving (10g, 49 Calories) contains:

5 Significant Nutrients	
Nutrient	DRI Per Serving (Daily Recommended Intake)
Omega-3 ALA	1097%
Omega 6 LA	34%
Phosphorus	14%
Copper	11%
Fiber	10%

34. Lentils

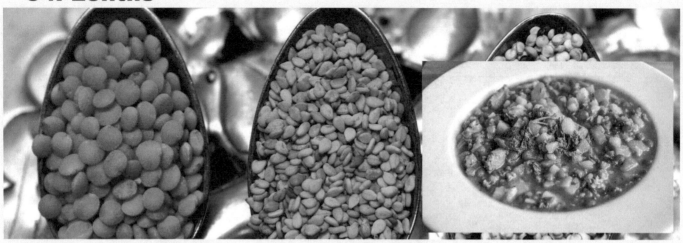

What are Lentils?

Lentils, small legumes from the Lens culinaris plant, are not only a staple in many cuisines but also offer substantial health benefits. Rich in folate, lentils contribute to DNA synthesis, cell division, and the formation of red blood cells, supporting overall growth and development. They are also a valuable source of iron, aiding in oxygen transport and energy metabolism, and are particularly important for individuals at risk of iron deficiency.

Lentils are packed with dietary fiber, promoting digestive health, regulating blood sugar levels, and providing a sense of fullness, aiding in weight management. Additionally, they contain a variety of vitamins and minerals, including potassium and magnesium, contributing to heart health and overall well-being.

Incorporating lentils into a balanced diet provides a nutrient-dense source of plant-based protein, fiber, and essential nutrients, making them a healthful and versatile choice for various culinary applications.

Top Diseases/Conditions

Lentils are identified as a top food for 39 of the Top 100 Diseases and Conditions. Of those, 3 Diseases and Conditions rank it as #1 (Golden Bullets), while 4 of them rank it between #2 and #10 (Silver Bullets).

3 Golden Bullets	Definition: #1 Top Food for each given condition (other than Water)
Gallstoness	Pregnancy
Gastritis	

4 Silver Bullets	Definition: Top 10 food for each given condition (but not #1)
Autism	Fibroids
Bipolar Disorder	Hemorrhoids

Nutrients?

One serving (96g, 112 Calories) contains:

12 Significant Nutrients	
Nutrient	DRI Per Serving (Daily Recommended Intake)
Vitamin B9 (Folate)	43%
Iron	40%
Copper	27%
Phosphorus	25%
Manganese	21%
Fiber	20%
Protein	15%
Vitamin B6	15%
Vitamin B5 (Pantothenic Acid)	13%
Vitamin B1 (Thiamine)	12%
Zinc	11%
Potassium	10%

35. Kidney Beans

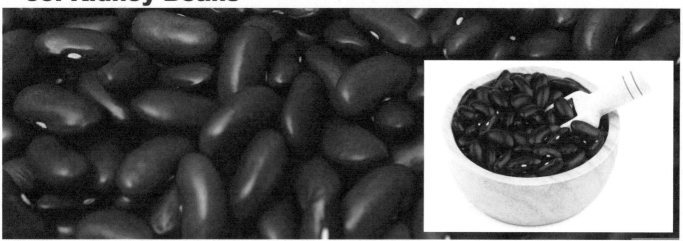

What are Kidney Beans?

Kidney beans, large reddish-brown legumes from the Phaseolus vulgaris plant, are not only a popular ingredient in various dishes but also offer notable health benefits. Rich in plant-based protein, kidney beans are an excellent source of essential amino acids, supporting muscle health and overall bodily functions. They are also packed with dietary fiber, promoting digestive health, regulating blood sugar levels, and contributing to weight management.

Kidney beans are a good source of complex carbohydrates, providing sustained energy. Additionally, they contain a range of vitamins and minerals, including folate, iron, and potassium, supporting various aspects of health, such as red blood cell formation, oxygen transport, and heart health.

Incorporating kidney beans into a balanced diet adds a nutrient-dense and versatile source of plant-based protein and essential nutrients, making them a healthy and flavorful choice for a wide range of culinary applications.

Top Diseases/Conditions

Kidney Beans are identified as a top food for 38 of the Top 100 Diseases and Conditions. Of those, 1 Diseases and Conditions rank it as #1 (Golden Bullets), while 4 of them rank it between #2 and #10 (Silver Bullets).

1 Golden Bullet	Definition: #1 Top Food for each given condition (other than Water)
Anemia of Chronic Disease	

4 Silver Bullets	Definition: Top 10 food for each given condition (but not #1)
ADHD	High Cholesterol
Chlamydia	Iron Deficiency Anemia

Nutrients?

One serving (92g, 77 Calories) contains:

5 Significant Nutrients	
Nutrient	DRI Per Serving (Daily Recommended Intake)
Sodium	18%
Iron	13%
Fiber	13%
Copper	12%
Phosphorus	12%

36. Collard Greens

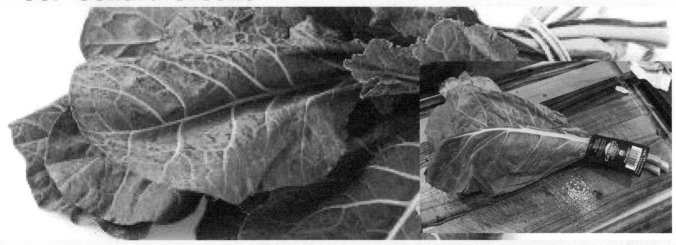

What are Collard Greens?

Collard greens, leafy vegetables from the Brassica oleracea family, are nutritional powerhouses known for their health benefits. Rich in vitamin K, collard greens support blood clotting, bone health, and cardiovascular function. They are also a good source of vitamin A, essential for vision, immune function, and skin health.

The presence of antioxidants, such as beta-carotene and flavonoids, contributes to the anti-inflammatory and potential anti-cancer properties of collard greens. Additionally, these greens provide dietary fiber, promoting digestive health, regulating blood sugar levels, and aiding in weight management.

Incorporating collard greens into a balanced diet adds a low-calorie, nutrient-dense option rich in vitamins, minerals, and antioxidants. Whether sautéed, steamed, or added to soups, collard greens offer a delicious and healthful addition to meals, supporting overall well-being.

Top Diseases/Conditions

Collard Greens are identified as a top food for 42 of the Top 100 Diseases and Conditions. Of those, 2 Diseases and Conditions rank it as #1 (Golden Bullets), while 5 of them rank it between #2 and #10 (Silver Bullets).

2 Golden Bullets	Definition: #1 Top Food for each given condition (other than Water)
Fibromyalgia	Osteoporosis

5 Silver Bullets	Definition: Top 10 food for each given condition (but not #1)
Acne	Inguinal Hernia
Cancer: Non-Hodgkin's Lymphoma	Osteoarthritis
Fibroids	

Nutrients?

One serving (36g, 11 Calories) contains:

4 Significant Nutrients	
Nutrient	DRI Per Serving (Daily Recommended Intake)
Vitamin K	153%
Vitamin A	80%
Vitamin B9 (Folate)	15%
Vitamin C	14%

37. Chickpeas

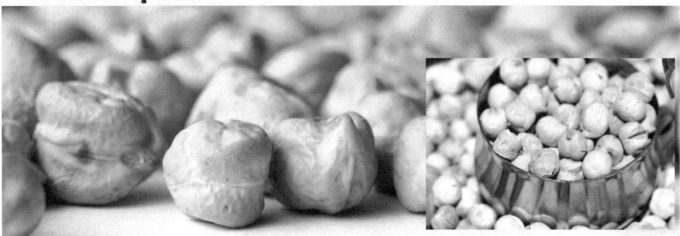

What are Chickpeas?

Chickpeas, also known as garbanzo beans, are legumes packed with nutritional benefits. Rich in vitamin B6, chickpeas play a vital role in brain development, immune function, and the synthesis of neurotransmitters. They are also a good source of manganese, supporting bone formation, collagen production, and antioxidant defense.

Chickpeas provide a well-balanced combination of protein, complex carbohydrates, and dietary fiber, contributing to satiety, blood sugar regulation, and digestive health. Their low glycemic index makes them suitable for individuals managing blood sugar levels.

The diverse nutrient profile of chickpeas makes them a valuable addition to a balanced diet, supporting overall well-being. Whether added to salads, soups, or blended into hummus, chickpeas offer a versatile and nutritious option, promoting sustained energy and providing essential vitamins and minerals for various bodily functions.

Top Diseases/Conditions

Chickpeas are identified as a top food for 46 of the Top 100 Diseases and Conditions. Of those, 2 Diseases and Conditions rank it as #1 (Golden Bullets), while 5 of them rank it between #2 and #10 (Silver Bullets).

2 Golden Bullets	Definition: #1 Top Food for each given condition (other than Water)
Anemia of Chronic Disease	Celiac Disease

5 Silver Bullets	Definition: Top 10 food for each given condition (but not #1)
ADHD	Iron Deficiency Anemia
Bipolar Disorder	Menopause
Inflammatory Bowel Disease	

Nutrients?

One serving (100g, 119 Calories) contains:

9 Significant Nutrients	
Nutrient	DRI Per Serving (Daily Recommended Intake)
Vitamin B6	38%
Manganese	26%
Copper	22%
Sodium	20%
Vitamin B9 (Folate)	17%
Iron	16%
Phosphorus	13%
Fiber	12%
Zinc	10%

38. Milk

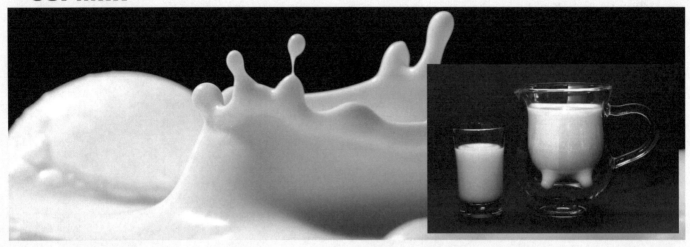

What is Milk?

Milk, derived from mammals like cows, is a nutrient-rich beverage with several health benefits. It is an excellent source of calcium, crucial for bone health, muscle function, and blood clotting. Vitamin B12 in dairy milk supports nerve function, red blood cell formation, and overall energy metabolism. Phosphorus, another essential mineral found in milk, is vital for bone and teeth health, kidney function, and cell repair.

Milk is also rich in vitamin B2 (riboflavin), necessary for energy production, cellular growth, and maintaining healthy skin. The combination of these nutrients in milk makes it a well-rounded option for promoting overall bone health, maintaining energy levels, and supporting various bodily functions.

Incorporating milk into a balanced diet provides a convenient and delicious way to ensure adequate intake of essential nutrients, contributing to overall well-being and nutritional requirements.

Top Diseases/Conditions

Milk is identified as a top food for 31 of the Top 100 Diseases and Conditions. Of those, 1 Diseases and Conditions rank it as #1 (Golden Bullets), while 9 of them rank it between #2 and #10 (Silver Bullets).

1 Golden Bullet	Definition: #1 Top Food for each given condition (other than Water)
Lumbar Radiculopathy	

9 Silver Bullets	Definition: Top 10 food for each given condition (but not #1)
Asthma	Osteoporosis
Cancer: Thyroid	Premenstrual Syndrome
Hyperthyroidism	Sleep Apnea
Hypothyroidism	Syncope
Oral / Dental Health	

Nutrients?

One serving (227g, 127 Calories) contains:

8 Significant Nutrients	
Nutrient	DRI Per Serving (Daily Recommended Intake)
Vitamin B12	37%
Phosphorus	36%
Vitamin B2 (Riboflavin)	34%
Calcium	32%
Protein	16%
Vitamin B5 (Pantothenic Acid)	15%
Potassium	12%
Selenium	11%

39. Onions

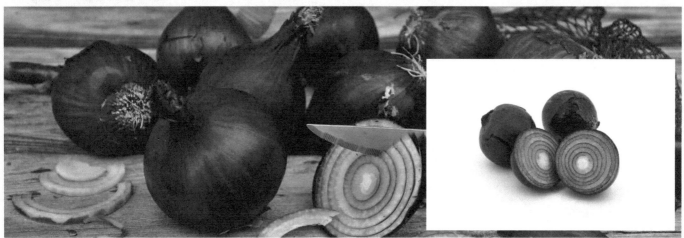

What are Onions?

Onions, flavorful bulbs from the Allium family, are not only culinary staples but also offer numerous health benefits. Rich in antioxidants, particularly quercetin, onions have anti-inflammatory properties and may contribute to heart health by reducing blood pressure and cholesterol levels. They contain vitamin C, supporting immune function and skin health, and are a good source of fiber, promoting digestive health and weight management.

Onions also contain sulfur compounds with potential anti-cancer properties and may support detoxification processes in the body. Additionally, they provide essential minerals like potassium and manganese, contributing to overall well-being.

Incorporating onions into a balanced diet adds depth of flavor and a range of nutrients, making them a versatile and healthful ingredient in various dishes while supporting numerous aspects of health.

Red onions are often considered more beneficial than other types of onions for several reasons, primarily related to their higher levels of antioxidants, particularly quercetin and anthocyanins. These compounds help protect the body against oxidative stress and may reduce the risk of chronic diseases such as heart disease and cancer. The antioxidants and flavonoids in red onions have anti-inflammatory effects, which can help reduce inflammation in the body and potentially lower the risk of inflammatory diseases.

Top Diseases/Conditions

Onions are identified as a top food for 18 of the Top 100 Diseases and Conditions. Of those, 1 Diseases and Conditions rank it as #1 (Golden Bullets), while 2 of them rank it between #2 and #10 (Silver Bullets).

1 Golden Bullet	Definition: #1 Top Food for each given condition (other than Water)
Allergies Rhinitis	

2 Silver Bullets	Definition: Top 10 food for each given condition (but not #1)
Brain Tumors	Rosacea

Nutrients?

One serving (148g, 59 Calories) contains:

3 Significant Nutrients	
Nutrient	DRI Per Serving (Daily Recommended Intake)
Vitamin B6	14%
Vitamin C	12%
Copper	10%

40. Swiss Chard

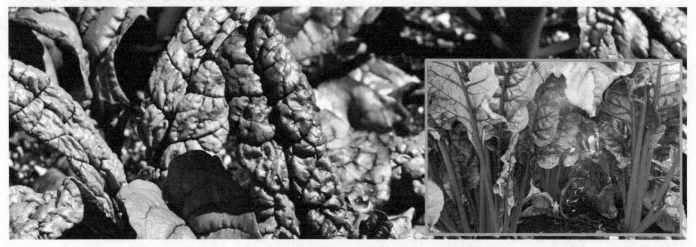

What is Swiss Chard?

Swiss chard, a leafy green vegetable from the Beta vulgaris family, is a nutritional powerhouse with various health benefits. Rich in vitamin K, Swiss chard supports blood clotting and bone health. While it doesn't contain significant amounts of vitamin D, it does provide essential nutrients like magnesium and vitamin A, promoting immune function and vision.

Swiss chard is a low-calorie food packed with antioxidants, such as beta-carotene and flavonoids, which have anti-inflammatory and potential anti-cancer properties. Its high fiber content supports digestive health, regulates blood sugar levels, and aids in weight management.

Incorporating Swiss chard into a balanced diet adds a burst of nutrients, offering versatility in salads, sautés, or smoothies. Its diverse nutrient profile contributes to overall well-being, making it a delicious and healthful choice for those seeking nutrient-rich greens in their meals.

Top Diseases/Conditions

Swiss Chard is identified as a top food for 34 of the Top 100 Diseases and Conditions. Of those, 5 of them rank it between #2 and #10 (Silver Bullets).

5 Silver Bullets	Definition: Top 10 food for each given condition (but not #1)
Acne	Oral / Dental Health
Migrain	Osteoarthritis
OCD	

Nutrients?

One serving (36g, 7 Calories) contains:

4 Significant Nutrients	
Nutrient	DRI Per Serving (Daily Recommended Intake)
Vitamin K	249%
Vitamin A	73%
Vitamin C	12%
Copper	11%

41. Cheese

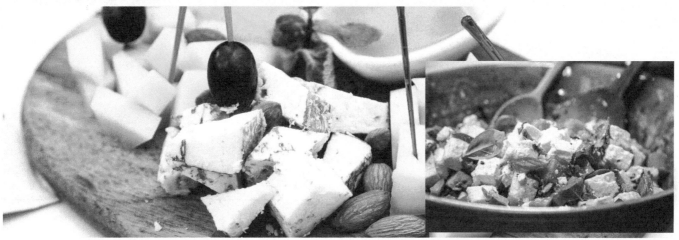

What is Cheese?

Cheese, a dairy product made from milk, is not only a delicious addition to many dishes but also provides essential nutrients. Rich in vitamin B12, cheese supports nerve function, red blood cell formation, and overall energy metabolism. It is also an excellent source of calcium, vital for bone health, muscle function, and blood clotting, as well as phosphorus, which contributes to bone and teeth strength, kidney function, and cell repair.

The combination of these nutrients in cheese makes it a nutritious choice for supporting overall bone health, preventing deficiencies, and maintaining optimal energy levels. However, moderation is key due to its calorie and fat content. Including cheese in a well-balanced diet adds a flavorful and nutrient-rich component, offering not only taste but also essential vitamins and minerals for various bodily functions.

Top Diseases/Conditions

Cheese is identified as a top food for 28 of the Top 100 Diseases and Conditions. Of those, 6 of them rank it between #2 and #10 (Silver Bullets).

6 Silver Bullets	Definition: Top 10 food for each given condition (but not #1)
Bipolar Disorder	Lumbar Radiculopathy
Cold Sores	Oral / Dental Health
Genital Herpes	Osteoporosis

Nutrients?

One serving (40g, 120 Calories) contains:

7 Significant Nutrients	
Nutrient	DRI Per Serving (Daily Recommended Intake)
Vitamin B12	38%
Phosphorus	20%
Calcium	20%
Sodium	17%
Protein	16%
Selenium	12%
Zinc	11%

42. Dark Chocolate

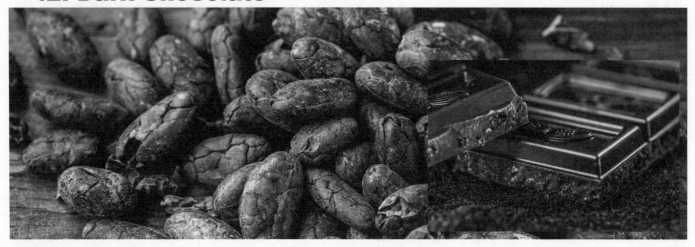

What is Dark Chocolate?

Dark chocolate, derived from cocoa beans, is a delectable treat that also offers several health benefits. Rich in copper, dark chocolate supports iron absorption, energy metabolism, and the formation of connective tissues. It is also a good source of iron, contributing to oxygen transport, immune function, and overall energy production.

Dark chocolate contains flavonoids, powerful antioxidants that may help improve heart health by reducing blood pressure and enhancing blood flow. Additionally, it has been associated with improved mood and cognitive function due to its content of compounds like theobromine and phenylethylamine.

Consuming dark chocolate in moderation provides a pleasurable way to incorporate essential minerals and antioxidants into a balanced diet. Opting for chocolate with higher cocoa content ensures a greater concentration of these beneficial compounds, offering a tasty and healthful indulgence for those with a sweet tooth.

Top Diseases/Conditions

Dark Chocolate is identified as a top food for 22 of the Top 100 Diseases and Conditions. Of those, 1 Diseases and Conditions rank it as #1 (Golden Bullets), while 3 of them rank it between #2 and #10 (Silver Bullets).

1 Golden Bullet	Definition: #1 Top Food for each given condition (other than Water)
Anxiety Disorder	

3 Silver Bullets	Definition: Top 10 food for each given condition (but not #1)
Alzheimer's/Dementia	Glaucoma
Bipolar Disorder	

Nutrients?

One serving (30g, 180 Calories) contains:

6 Significant Nutrients	
Nutrient	DRI Per Serving (Daily Recommended Intake)
Copper	60%
Iron	45%
Manganese	25%
Magnesium	16%
Phosphorus	13%
"Good" Fat	10%

43. Grass-Fed Beef

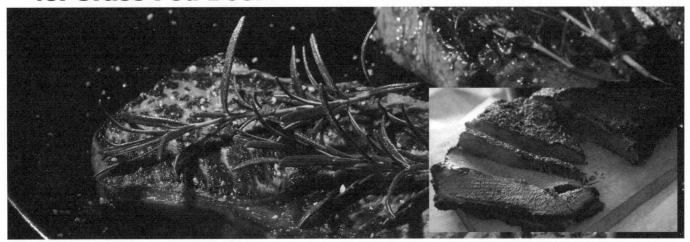

What is Grass-Fed Beef?

Grass-fed beef comes from cattle that primarily graze on natural pasture, offering nutritional advantages. Rich in vitamin B12, grass-fed beef supports nerve function, red blood cell formation, and overall energy metabolism. It is also a high-quality source of protein, essential for muscle development, repair, and immune function. Additionally, grass-fed beef provides zinc, a mineral crucial for immune support, wound healing, and DNA synthesis.

Compared to conventionally raised beef, grass-fed varieties often contain higher levels of beneficial nutrients, including omega-3 fatty acids and antioxidants. These nutritional differences are attributed to the cattle's natural diet of grass, contributing to potential heart health benefits and reduced inflammation.

Incorporating grass-fed beef into a balanced diet offers a nutrient-dense protein source with potential additional health advantages. Choosing grass-fed options aligns with sustainable and ethical farming practices, providing consumers with a choice that supports both personal health and environmental well-being.

Top Diseases/Conditions

Grass-Fed Beef is identified as a top food for 28 of the Top 100 Diseases and Conditions. Of those, 1 Diseases and Conditions rank it as #1 (Golden Bullets), while 7 of them rank it between #2 and #10 (Silver Bullets).

1 Golden Bullet	Definition: #1 Top Food for each given condition (other than Water)
Anemia of Chronic Disease	

7 Silver Bullets	Definition: Top 10 food for each given condition (but not #1)
Acne	OCD
Cancer: Thyroid	Shingles (Herpes Zoster)
Hypothyroidism	Syncope
Iron Deficiency Anemia	

Nutrients?

One serving (85g, 163 Calories) contains:

12 Significant Nutrients	
Nutrient	DRI Per Serving (Daily Recommended Intake)
Vitamin B12	71%
Zinc	35%
Protein	29%
Vitamin B6	26%
Vitamin B3 (Niacin)	26%
Selenium	22%
Iron	21%
Phosphorus	21%
Vitamin B2 (Riboflavin)	13%
Choline	10%
"Good" Fat	10%
Vitamin B5 (Pantothenic Acid)	10%

44. Local Honey

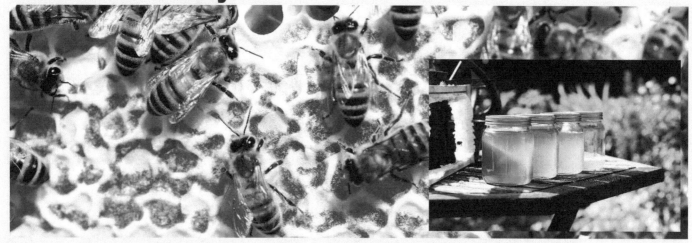

What is Local Honey?

Local honey is honey produced by bees in close proximity to where it is consumed. Unlike commercially processed honey, local honey is typically minimally filtered and may contain traces of local pollen. Consuming local honey is often associated with potential health benefits. Some believe that regular intake of local honey may help alleviate seasonal allergies, as exposure to local pollen in small amounts could potentially desensitize the immune system.

Additionally, local honey is a natural sweetener with antimicrobial properties, aiding in wound healing and providing a healthier alternative to refined sugars. Rich in antioxidants, enzymes, and trace minerals, local honey can contribute to overall well-being. However, it's important to note that moderation is key due to its calorie content. Supporting local beekeepers by choosing local honey also promotes sustainable agriculture and biodiversity.

Top Diseases/Conditions

Local Honey is identified as a top food for 8 of the Top 100 Diseases and Conditions. Of those, 2 Diseases and Conditions rank it as #1 (Golden Bullets), while 1 of them rank it between #2 and #10 (Silver Bullets).

2 Golden Bullets	Definition: #1 Top Food for each given condition (other than Water)
Allergies Rhinitis	Streptococcal Pharyngitis

1 Silver Bullet	Definition: Top 10 food for each given condition (but not #1)
Common Cold / Virus	

Nutrients?

One serving (21g, 64 Calories) contains no nutrients that are at least 10% DRI.

45. Quinoa

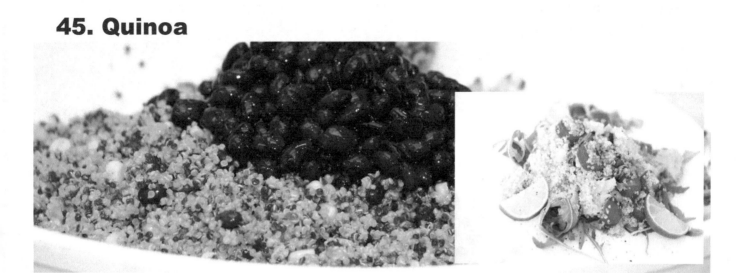

What is Quinoa?

Quinoa is a nutrient-dense, gluten-free grain-like seed originating from South America. It is a rich source of essential minerals, including manganese, which supports bone health, metabolism, and antioxidant defenses. Quinoa also contains copper, vital for iron metabolism, collagen formation, and overall immune function. The presence of phosphorus in quinoa contributes to bone and teeth health, while iron supports oxygen transport, energy metabolism, and red blood cell formation.

Quinoa stands out as a complete protein, containing all nine essential amino acids, making it an excellent plant-based protein source for vegetarians and vegans. Its high fiber content supports digestive health and helps regulate blood sugar levels.

Incorporating quinoa into a balanced diet adds a versatile, nutritious component, offering a range of essential nutrients and health benefits. This ancient grain contributes to overall well-being, making it a popular choice for those seeking a wholesome and diverse dietary option.

Top Diseases/Conditions

Quinoa is identified as a top food for 31 of the Top 100 Diseases and Conditions. Of those, 3 Diseases and Conditions rank it as #1 (Golden Bullets), while 4 of them rank it between #2 and #10 (Silver Bullets).

3 Golden Bullets	Definition: #1 Top Food for each given condition (other than Water)
Celiac Disease	Stroke/TIA
Kidney Stone	

4 Silver Bullets	Definition: Top 10 food for each given condition (but not #1)
Bipolar Disorder	Inguinal Hernia
Brain Tumors	Rheumatoid Arthritis

Nutrients?

One serving (1/6 Cup Uncooked, 28g, 111 Calories) or (1/2 Cup Cooked, 93g, 111 Calories) contains:

11 Significant Nutrients	
Nutrient	DRI Per Serving (Daily Recommended Intake)
Manganese	38%
Copper	27%
Phosphorus	27%
Iron	24%
Magnesium	20%
Vitamin B9 (Folate)	19%
Vitamin B6	15%
Vitamin B1 (Thiamine)	12%
Zinc	12%
Protein	11%
Vitamin B2 (Riboflavin)	10%

46. Turkey

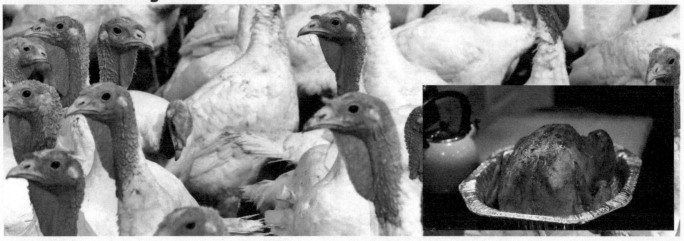

What is Turkey?

Turkey, particularly the skinless breast, is a lean and nutritious meat with various health benefits. It is a great source of vitamin B6, essential for metabolism, immune function, and neurotransmitter synthesis. The presence of selenium in turkey supports antioxidant defenses, thyroid function, and immune health. High in protein, turkey breast is crucial for muscle development, repair, and overall tissue maintenance. Additionally, turkey provides niacin, promoting heart health and aiding in energy metabolism.

Choosing skinless turkey breast is a healthier option as it reduces saturated fat intake. This lean protein source is associated with weight management and cardiovascular health. The amino acid tryptophan in turkey contributes to the production of serotonin, supporting mood regulation and relaxation.

Incorporating skinless turkey breast into a balanced diet offers a nutrient-dense, low-fat protein option with a range of essential vitamins and minerals, contributing to overall well-being and supporting various bodily functions.

Top Diseases/Conditions

Turkey is identified as a top food for 31 of the Top 100 Diseases and Conditions. Of those, 1 Diseases and Conditions rank it as #1 (Golden Bullets), while 3 of them rank it between #2 and #10 (Silver Bullets).

1 Golden Bullet	Definition: #1 Top Food for each given condition (other than Water)
Kidney Stone	

3 Silver Bullets	Definition: Top 10 food for each given condition (but not #1)
Alopecia Areata	Insomnia
Autism	

Nutrients?

One serving (85g, 94 Calories) contains:

10 Significant Nutrients	
Nutrient	DRI Per Serving (Daily Recommended Intake)
Vitamin B6	39%
Selenium	38%
Protein	37%
Vitamin B3 (Niacin)	33%
Phosphorus	25%
Vitamin B12	16%
Iron	13%
Vitamin B5 (Pantothenic Acid)	12%
Copper	12%
Zinc	10%

47. Bell Peppers

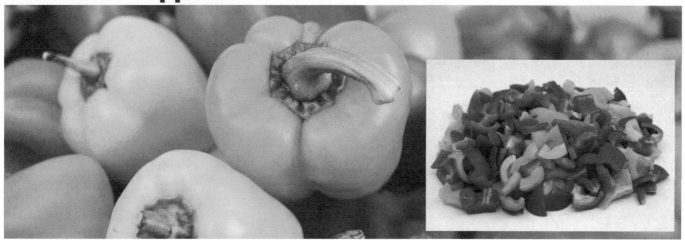

What is Bell Peppers?

Bell peppers are colorful and nutritious vegetables that come in various hues, such as red, green, and yellow. They are particularly rich in vitamin C, a powerful antioxidant essential for immune function, collagen synthesis, and skin health. The high vitamin C content in bell peppers supports the body's defense against oxidative stress and aids in the absorption of non-heme iron from plant-based foods.

Beyond vitamin C, bell peppers contain a variety of other vitamins, including A and B6, along with minerals like folate. Their low calorie and high fiber content make them a valuable addition to a balanced diet, supporting weight management and digestive health.

Incorporating bell peppers into meals not only adds vibrant color and flavor but also provides a nutrient-packed option that contributes to overall well-being and helps meet daily vitamin and mineral requirements.

Top Diseases/Conditions

Bell Peppers are identified as a top food for 22 of the Top 100 Diseases and Conditions. Of those, 5 Diseases and Conditions rank it as #1 (Golden Bullets), while 4 of them rank it between #2 and #10 (Silver Bullets).

5 Golden Bullets	Definition: #1 Top Food for each given condition (other than Water)
Cataracts	Kidney Stone
Chronic Kidney Disease	Peptic Ulcer
Influenza	

4 Silver Bullets	Definition: Top 10 food for each given condition (but not #1)
Cold Sores	Mononucleosis
Genital Herpes	Shingles (Herpes Zoster)

Nutrients?

One serving (148g, 40 Calories) contains:

5 Significant Nutrients	
Nutrient	DRI Per Serving (Daily Recommended Intake)
Vitamin C	301%
Vitamin B6	18%
Copper	18%
Vitamin A	10%
Vitamin B9 (Folate)	10%

48. Cherries

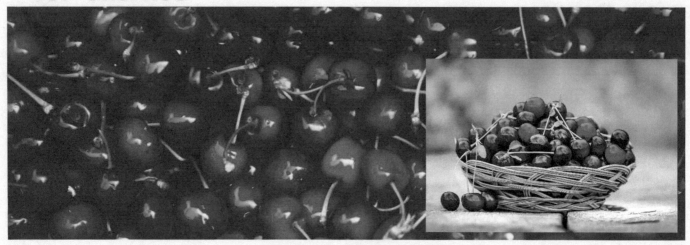

What are Cherries?

Cherries are delicious and nutritious fruits that offer a range of health benefits. Rich in vitamin C, cherries contribute to immune system support, collagen synthesis, and antioxidant defenses, promoting overall well-being. The presence of copper in cherries further supports the immune system and aids in the formation of connective tissues, bones, and red blood cells.

Beyond these nutrients, cherries contain bioactive compounds like anthocyanins, which possess anti-inflammatory and antioxidant properties. These compounds are associated with various health benefits, including reducing oxidative stress and inflammation in the body. Cherries may also have potential benefits for joint health and sleep due to their natural melatonin content.

Incorporating cherries into a balanced diet provides a flavorful and healthful addition, offering a sweet and nutrient-rich option that contributes to overall health and may have positive effects on various aspects of well-being.

Top Diseases/Conditions

Cherries are identified as a top food for 12 of the Top 100 Diseases and Conditions. Of those, 2 Diseases and Conditions rank it as #1 (Golden Bullets), while 2 of them rank it between #2 and #10 (Silver Bullets).

2 Golden Bullets	Definition: #1 Top Food for each given condition (other than Water)
Gout	Sleep Apnea

2 Silver Bullets	Definition: Top 10 food for each given condition (but not #1)
Contact Dermatitis	Insomnia

Nutrients?

One serving (140g, 88 Calories) contains:

2 Significant Nutrients	
Nutrient	DRI Per Serving (Daily Recommended Intake)
Copper	11%
Vitamin C	11%

49. Limes

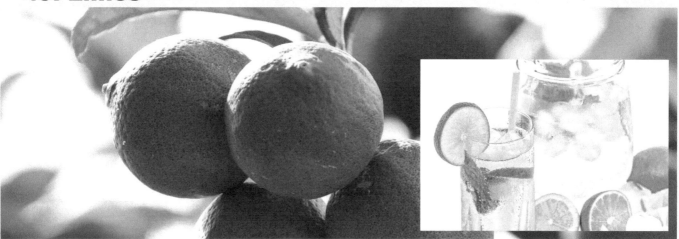

What are Limes?

Limes are citrus fruits packed with health benefits. Rich in vitamin C, limes support immune function, collagen synthesis, and antioxidant defenses, contributing to overall well-being. Their flavonoid content may have anti-inflammatory and anticancer properties, offering potential health advantages. Limes also provide a good dose of potassium, aiding in heart health, blood pressure regulation, and muscle function.

The citric acid in limes may promote digestive health and assist in the absorption of minerals. Additionally, their low calorie and high fiber content make limes a weight-friendly snack that supports digestive regularity.

Incorporating limes into a balanced diet not only adds refreshing flavor but also provides a nutrient-rich option with various vitamins and antioxidants. Whether used in beverages, salads, or as a garnish, limes contribute to a tasty and healthful diet.

Top Diseases/Conditions

Limes are identified as a top food for 19 of the Top 100 Diseases and Conditions. Of those, 1 of them rank it between #2 and #10 (Silver Bullets).

1 Silver Bullet	Definition: Top 10 food for each given condition (but not #1)
Aortic Aneurysm	

Nutrients?

One serving (67g, 20 Calories) contains:

1 Significant Nutrient	
Nutrient	DRI Per Serving (Daily Recommended Intake)
Vitamin C	22%

50. Cabbage

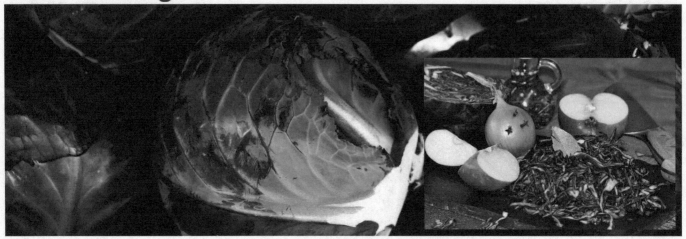

What is Cabbage?

Cabbage is a cruciferous vegetable with numerous health benefits. Rich in vitamin C, cabbage supports immune function, collagen synthesis, and antioxidant defenses, contributing to overall well-being. Its folate content is essential for DNA synthesis and repair, making it crucial for cell division and growth. Cabbage also contains fiber, promoting digestive health and aiding in weight management.

Beyond these nutrients, cabbage is known for its phytochemicals, including glucosinolates, which may have anti-cancer properties. The high water content in cabbage contributes to hydration and satiety, making it a valuable addition to a weight-conscious diet.

Incorporating cabbage into meals, whether raw in salads or cooked in stir-fries, provides a low-calorie, nutrient-dense option. Its versatility, along with its nutritional profile, makes cabbage a healthful choice for supporting various bodily functions and contributing to overall health.

Top Diseases/Conditions

Cabbage is identified as a top food for 22 of the Top 100 Diseases and Conditions. Of those, 3 Diseases and Conditions rank it as #1 (Golden Bullets), while 1 of them rank it between #2 and #10 (Silver Bullets).

3 Golden Bullets	Definition: #1 Top Food for each given condition (other than Water)
Chronic Kidney Disease	Peptic Ulcer
Osteoporosis	

1 Silver Bullet	Definition: Top 10 food for each given condition (but not #1)
Fibroids	

Nutrients?

One serving (84g, 20 Calories) contains:

2 Significant Nutrients	
Nutrient	DRI Per Serving (Daily Recommended Intake)
Vitamin C	48%
Vitamin B9 (Folate)	12%

51. Cantaloupe

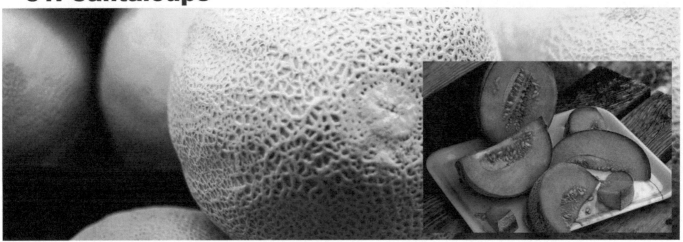

What is Cantaloupe?

Cantaloupe is a delicious and hydrating melon with notable health benefits. It is a rich source of both vitamin A and vitamin C. Vitamin A is essential for vision, immune function, and skin health, while vitamin C supports immune function, collagen synthesis, and acts as a powerful antioxidant.

Cantaloupe's high water content contributes to hydration and helps maintain optimal bodily functions. The fruit also contains dietary fiber, aiding in digestion and promoting a feeling of fullness.

In addition to its vitamins, cantaloupe contains antioxidants like beta-carotene, which may have protective effects against chronic diseases. The natural sweetness and refreshing nature of cantaloupe make it a satisfying and healthful choice for snacks, breakfast, or desserts, providing a tasty way to meet daily nutrient requirements and contribute to overall well-being.

Top Diseases/Conditions

Cantaloupe is identified as a top food for 16 of the Top 100 Diseases and Conditions. Of those, 1 Diseases and Conditions rank it as #1 (Golden Bullets), while 2 of them rank it between #2 and #10 (Silver Bullets).

1 Golden Bullet	Definition: #1 Top Food for each given condition (other than Water)
GERD / Heartburn	

2 Silver Bullets	Definition: Top 10 food for each given condition (but not #1)
Gastroenteritis	Syncope

Nutrients?

One serving (177g, 60 Calories) contains:

4 Significant Nutrients	
Nutrient	DRI Per Serving (Daily Recommended Intake)
Vitamin A	200%
Vitamin C	72%
Potassium	14%
Copper	11%

52. Green Tea

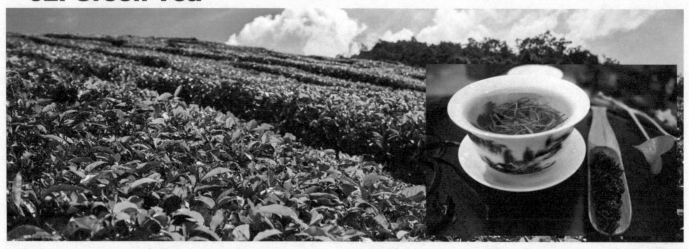

What is Green Tea?

Green tea is a popular beverage made from Camellia sinensis leaves and is known for its numerous health benefits. Rich in antioxidants, particularly catechins like epigallocatechin gallate (EGCG), green tea has potential anti-inflammatory and anticancer properties. Regular consumption is linked to improved heart health, as it may help lower cholesterol levels and reduce blood pressure.

The presence of L-theanine in green tea provides a calming effect, promoting relaxation and mental alertness. Additionally, green tea is associated with weight management, aiding in metabolism and fat oxidation. Its potential to enhance brain function and lower the risk of neurodegenerative diseases adds to its appeal.

With relatively low caffeine content compared to coffee, green tea offers a hydrating and health-promoting alternative. Its diverse benefits make it a popular choice for those seeking a refreshing beverage that positively contributes to overall well-being.

Top Diseases/Conditions

Green Tea is identified as a top food for 29 of the Top 100 Diseases and Conditions. Of those, 2 Diseases and Conditions rank it as #1 (Golden Bullets), while 2 of them rank it between #2 and #10 (Silver Bullets).

2 Golden Bullets	Definition: #1 Top Food for each given condition (other than Water)
Cancer: Breast	Influenza

2 Silver Bullets	Definition: Top 10 food for each given condition (but not #1)
Mononucleosis	Parkinsons

Nutrients?

One serving (227g, 2 Calories) contains:

1 Significant Nutrient	
Nutrient	DRI Per Serving (Daily Recommended Intake)
Manganese	22%

53. Pumpkin Seeds

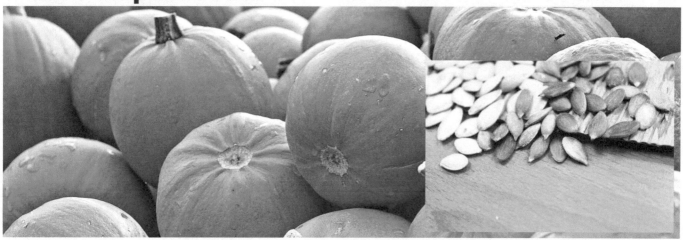

What are Pumpkin Seeds?

Pumpkin seeds, also known as pepitas, are nutrient-dense and offer a range of health benefits. Rich in iron, they support oxygen transport in the blood and prevent iron-deficiency anemia. The presence of phosphorus contributes to bone health, while copper aids in iron absorption and enzyme function. Pumpkin seeds are also a good source of magnesium, crucial for muscle and nerve function, blood pressure regulation, and bone health.

Additionally, these seeds contain omega-6 fatty acids, promoting heart health and reducing inflammation. Manganese in pumpkin seeds supports bone formation and antioxidant defenses. The seeds are a convenient and tasty snack that can be easily incorporated into various dishes, salads, or enjoyed on their own, providing a nutrient-rich option with a diverse profile of minerals that positively impact overall well-being.

Top Diseases/Conditions

Green Tea are identified as a top food for 26 of the Top 100 Diseases and Conditions. Of those, 1 Diseases and Conditions rank it as #1 (Golden Bullets), while 1 of them rank it between #2 and #10 (Silver Bullets).

1 Golden Bullet	Definition: #1 Top Food for each given condition (other than Water)
Hypertension	

1 Silver Bullet	Definition: Top 10 food for each given condition (but not #1)
Raynaud's Syndrome	

Nutrients?

One serving (28g, 151 Calories) contains:

10 Significant Nutrients	
Nutrient	DRI Per Serving (Daily Recommended Intake)
Iron	53%
Phosphorus	47%
Copper	44%
Magnesium	36%
Manganese	35%
Omega 6 LA	34%
"Good" Fat	23%
Zinc	19%
Protein	12%
Vitamin K	12%

54. Squash

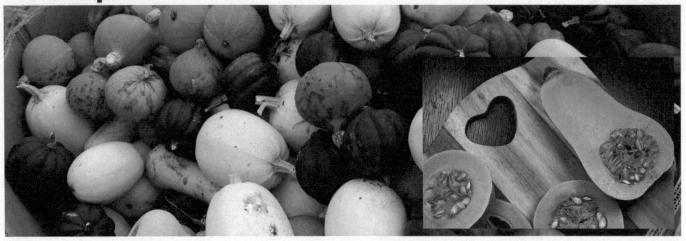

What is Squash?

Squash, most notably varieties like acorn and butternut, is a nutrient-packed vegetable with notable health benefits. Rich in vitamin A, squash supports vision, immune function, and skin health. The presence of beta-carotene, a precursor to vitamin A, gives squash its vibrant color and contributes to its antioxidant properties.

Squash is low in calories and high in dietary fiber, promoting digestive health and aiding in weight management. It also provides essential minerals like potassium, important for heart health and blood pressure regulation. The complex carbohydrates in squash release energy slowly, helping maintain stable blood sugar levels.

Acorn and butternut squash are versatile ingredients that can be roasted, pureed, or used in various recipes, making them a delicious and healthful addition to meals. Incorporating squash into your diet offers a tasty way to obtain essential nutrients and contribute to overall well-being.

Top Diseases/Conditions

Squash is identified as a top food for 21 of the Top 100 Diseases and Conditions. Of those, 3 of them rank it between #2 and #10 (Silver Bullets).

3 Silver Bullets	Definition: Top 10 food for each given condition (but not #1)
COPD	Plantar Warts
Diverticulitis	

Nutrients?

One serving (98g, 44 Calories) contains:

4 Significant Nutrients	
Nutrient	DRI Per Serving (Daily Recommended Intake)
Vitamin A	347%
Vitamin C	23%
Vitamin B6	11%
Potassium	10%

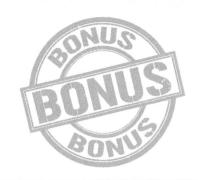

Healthiest Squash					
Type	Calories per serving	Percent of Daily DRI			
		Vitamin A	Vitamin C	Vitamin B6	Potassium
Butternut	44	347%	23%	11%	10%
Pumpkin	25	278%	10%	5%	10%
Acorn	39	12%	12%	12%	10%
Zucchini	17	7%	20%	12%	8%

Best   2nd Best

55. Sauerkraut

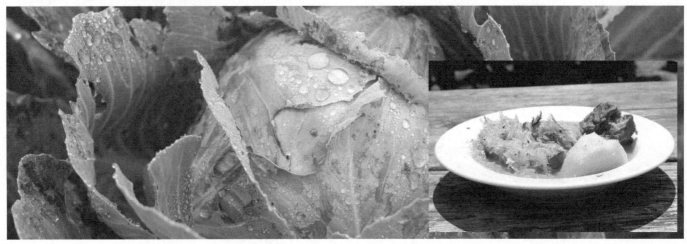

What is Sauerkraut?

Sauerkraut is a fermented cabbage dish that undergoes a natural fermentation process, creating a tangy flavor and numerous health benefits. While sauerkraut itself is not particularly high in iron, the fermentation process enhances nutrient absorption, potentially increasing iron bioavailability. It is, however, a rich source of vitamin C, which enhances non-heme iron absorption and supports the immune system.

Sauerkraut, as well as Kimchi, is a natural source of probiotics, beneficial bacteria that promote gut health by aiding digestion and supporting a balanced microbiome. The fermentation process also produces various bioactive compounds, including organic acids and phytochemicals, which may have anti-inflammatory and antioxidant effects.

Incorporating sauerkraut into your diet as a condiment or side dish provides a flavorful way to introduce probiotics and essential nutrients. Its potential to support digestive health and boost the immune system makes sauerkraut a healthful addition to a well-rounded diet.

Top Diseases/Conditions

Sauerkraut is identified as a top food for 12 of the Top 100 Diseases and Conditions. Of those, 1 of them rank it between #2 and #10 (Silver Bullets).

1 Silver Bullet	Definition: Top 10 food for each given condition (but not #1)
Autism	

Nutrients?

One serving (236g, 45 Calories) contains:

10 Significant Nutrients	
Nutrient	DRI Per Serving (Daily Recommended Intake)
Sodium	104%
Iron	44%
Vitamin C	39%
Vitamin K	26%
Vitamin B6	23%
Copper	22%
Fiber	18%
Manganese	17%
Vitamin B9 (Folate)	14%
Potassium	12%

56. Seaweed

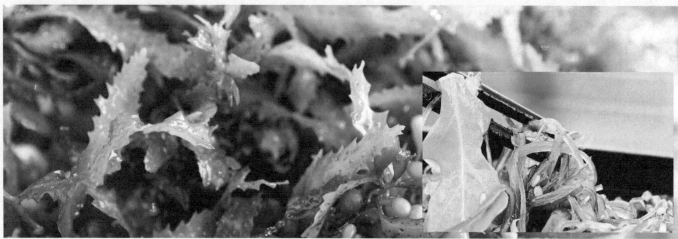

What is Seaweed?

Seaweed is a diverse group of marine algae that has been a staple in many Asian cuisines for centuries. It comes in various forms, such as nori, kelp, and wakame, and is rich in essential nutrients, making it a healthy addition to the diet. Seaweed is a notable source of iodine, crucial for thyroid function and hormone production.

Beyond iodine, seaweed provides a spectrum of vitamins, minerals, and antioxidants, including vitamin K, folate, magnesium, and iron. It is low in calories and carbohydrates while being a rich source of fiber, aiding in digestive health. The presence of bioactive compounds, such as fucoidans and phlorotannins, may contribute to antioxidant, anti-inflammatory, and anti-cancer properties.

Incorporating seaweed into meals, whether in sushi, salads, or soups, offers a nutrient-dense option with unique flavors and potential health benefits, supporting overall well-being.

Top Diseases/Conditions

Seaweed is identified as a top food for 18 of the Top 100 Diseases and Conditions. Of those, 2 Diseases and Conditions rank it as #1 (Golden Bullets), while 3 of them rank it between #2 and #10 (Silver Bullets).

2 Golden Bullets	Definition: #1 Top Food for each given condition (other than Water)
Hyperthyroidism	Hypothyroidism

3 Silver Bullets	Definition: Top 10 food for each given condition (but not #1)
Autism	OCD
Cancer: Thyroid	

Nutrients?

One serving (10g Dried, 5 Calories) contains no nutrients (that are included in this book) that are at least 10% DRI. However, it does contain Iodine, at a rate of 155% DRI per serving!

57. Potatoes

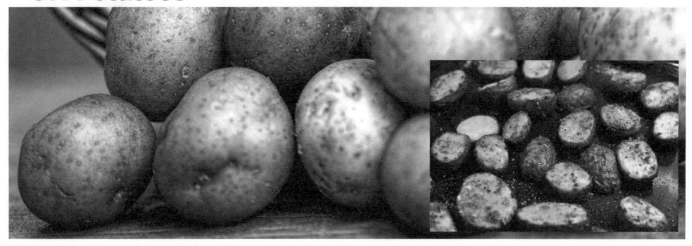

What are Potatoes?

Potatoes, including red varieties, are versatile and nutrient-rich vegetables. They are a good source of vitamin B6, essential for brain development, nerve function, and the formation of red blood cells. Vitamin B6 also plays a role in metabolizing proteins and maintaining hormonal balance.

Red potatoes, in particular, contain vitamin C, an antioxidant that supports immune function, collagen synthesis, and acts as a protective agent against oxidative stress. Potatoes also provide essential minerals like potassium, vital for heart health and blood pressure regulation.

While often associated with carbohydrates, potatoes contribute to a balanced diet when prepared in a healthful manner. They are a good source of complex carbohydrates and fiber, promoting digestive health and providing sustained energy. Including a variety of potatoes in your diet offers a delicious and nutritious way to obtain essential vitamins and minerals, supporting overall well-being.

Top Diseases/Conditions

Potatoes are identified as a top food for 18 of the Top 100 Diseases and Conditions. Of those, 1 of them rank it between #2 and #10 (Silver Bullets).

1 Silver Bullet	Definition: Top 10 food for each given condition (but not #1)
Diverticulitis	

Nutrients?

One serving (148g, 114 Calories) contains:

9 Significant Nutrients	
Nutrient	DRI Per Serving (Daily Recommended Intake)
Vitamin B6	34%
Vitamin C	32%
Potassium	18%
Copper	18%
Iron	15%
Phosphorus	12%
Manganese	10%
Vitamin B1 (Thiamine)	10%
Vitamin B3 (Niacin)	10%

58. Pineapple

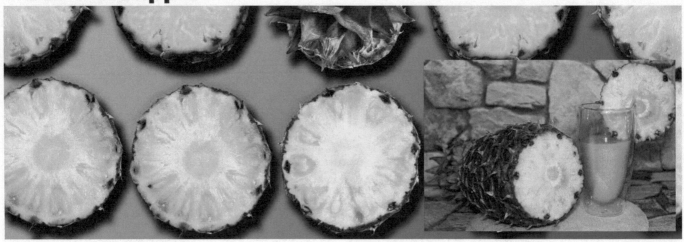

What is Pineapple?

Pineapples are tropical fruits known for their sweet and tangy flavor, offering a range of health benefits. Rich in vitamin C, pineapples contribute to immune system function, collagen synthesis, and antioxidant defenses. Vitamin C also supports skin health and aids in wound healing.

Additionally, pineapples contain manganese, a trace mineral important for bone formation, metabolism, and antioxidant enzyme function. Manganese also plays a role in collagen production, contributing to connective tissue health.

Beyond their nutrient content, pineapples contain bromelain, an enzyme with anti-inflammatory properties that may aid in digestion. The fruit's natural sweetness makes it a delicious and refreshing addition to various dishes and snacks.

Incorporating pineapples into your diet provides a flavorful way to obtain essential vitamins, minerals, and enzymes, contributing to overall well-being and supporting various bodily functions.

Top Diseases/Conditions

Pineapples are identified as a top food for 9 of the Top 100 Diseases and Conditions. Of those, 1 Diseases and Conditions rank it as #1 (Golden Bullets), while 1 of them rank it between #2 and #10 (Silver Bullets).

1 Golden Bullet	Definition: #1 Top Food for each given condition (other than Water)
HIV	

1 Silver Bullet	Definition: Top 10 food for each given condition (but not #1)
Tinnitus	

Nutrients?

One serving (112g, 56 Calories) contains:

4 Significant Nutrients	
Nutrient	DRI Per Serving *(Daily Recommended Intake)*
Vitamin C	60%
Manganese	45%
Copper	14%
Vitamin B6	10%

59. Whole Wheat

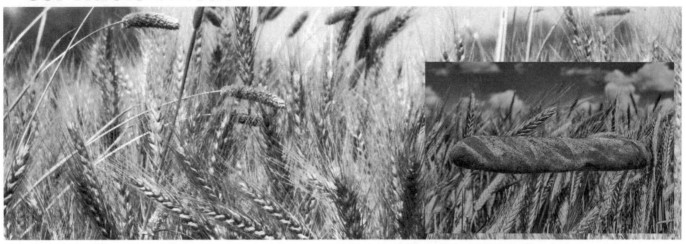

What is Whole Wheat?

Whole wheat refers to grains that retain all three parts of the kernel—the bran, germ, and endosperm—offering a more nutrient-dense option compared to refined grains. It is a rich source of manganese, a mineral that supports bone health, metabolism, and antioxidant defenses. Manganese also plays a role in collagen formation and wound healing.

Selenium is another essential mineral found in whole wheat, contributing to antioxidant enzyme function, thyroid health, and immune system support. Whole wheat's fiber content aids in digestion, helps regulate blood sugar levels, and promotes heart health.

Choosing whole wheat products over refined grains provides a more comprehensive array of nutrients, including B vitamins and fiber. The complex carbohydrates in whole wheat release energy gradually, providing sustained fuel for the body. Incorporating whole wheat into your diet offers a healthful option that supports overall well-being and contributes to a balanced nutrient intake.

Top Diseases/Conditions

Whole Wheat is identified as a top food for 12 of the Top 100 Diseases and Conditions. Of those, 2 of them rank it between #2 and #10 (Silver Bullets).

2 Silver Bullets	Definition: Top 10 food for each given condition (but not #1)
Diverticulitis	Tuberculosis (TB)

Nutrients?

One serving (36g, 37 Calories) contains:

2 Significant Nutrients	
Nutrient	DRI Per Serving (Daily Recommended Intake)
Manganese	18%
Selenium	14%

Notes
Typical serving is ½ Cup Cooked, 2/9 Cup Dry

60. Turmeric Root

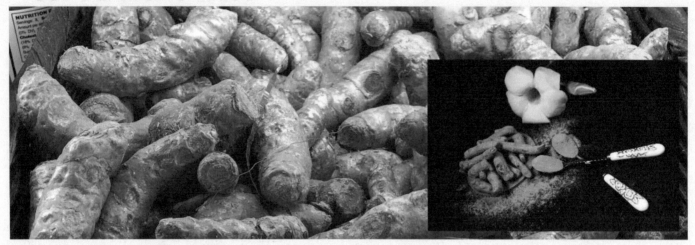

What is Turmeric Root?

Turmeric root, derived from the Curcuma longa plant, is renowned for its vibrant yellow color and numerous health benefits. Turmeric is a good source of manganese, an essential trace mineral involved in bone formation, metabolism, and antioxidant defenses. Manganese also plays a role in collagen production and wound healing.

The active compound in turmeric, curcumin, possesses potent anti-inflammatory and antioxidant properties. It may contribute to reducing inflammation, supporting joint health, and potentially offering protection against chronic diseases. Turmeric has been traditionally used in various cuisines and Ayurvedic medicine for its potential medicinal properties.

Incorporating turmeric into your diet, whether in curries, teas, or as a supplement, provides a flavorful way to introduce a bioactive compound with potential health benefits, supporting overall well-being and offering a natural approach to health maintenance.

Top Diseases/Conditions

Turmeric Root is identified as a top food for 25 of the Top 100 Diseases and Conditions. Of those, 1 Diseases and Conditions rank it as #1 (Golden Bullets), while 5 of them rank it between #2 and #10 (Silver Bullets).

1 Golden Bullet	Definition: #1 Top Food for each given condition (other than Water)
Peptic Ulcer	

5 Silver Bullets	Definition: Top 10 food for each given condition (but not #1)
Gastritis	Rheumatoid Arthritis
Pelvic Inflammatory Disease	Streptococcal Pharyngitis
Pneumonia	

Nutrients?

One serving (7g, 24 Calories) contains:

2 Significant Nutrients	
Nutrient	DRI Per Serving (Daily Recommended Intake)
Iron	35%
Manganese	22%

61. Barley

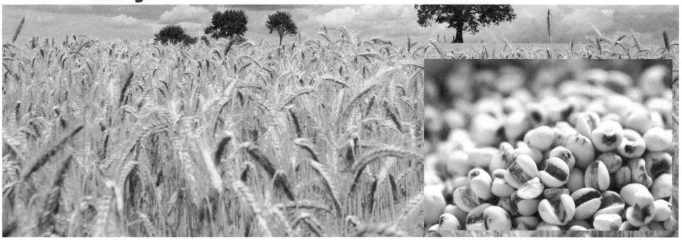

What is Barley?

Barley, specifically hulled barley, is a nutritious whole grain that has been a dietary staple for centuries. Unlike refined grains, hulled barley retains its outer bran layer and germ, providing a rich source of fiber, vitamins, and minerals. This minimally processed form of barley contributes to overall health in several ways.

Hulled barley is an excellent source of dietary fiber, promoting digestive health by supporting regular bowel movements and preventing constipation. The fiber content also aids in managing blood sugar levels and promoting a feeling of fullness, making it a valuable component for weight management.

In addition to fiber, hulled barley contains essential nutrients such as manganese, selenium, and B vitamins, which play roles in metabolism, antioxidant defense, and overall well-being. Including hulled barley in your diet provides a wholesome and versatile option, offering a range of health benefits through its nutrient-rich composition.

Top Diseases/Conditions

Barley is identified as a top food for 17 of the Top 100 Diseases and Conditions. Of those, 2 Diseases and Conditions rank it as #1 (Golden Bullets).

2 Golden Bullets	Definition: #1 Top Food for each given condition (other than Water)
Peripheral Arterial Disease	Rosacea

Nutrients?

One serving (44g, 156 Calories) contains:

12 Significant Nutrients	
Nutrient	DRI Per Serving (Daily Recommended Intake)
Manganese	37%
Selenium	30%
Copper	24%
Vitamin B1 (Thiamine)	24%
Fiber	20%
Iron	20%
Phosphorus	17%
Magnesium	14%
Vitamin B3 (Niacin)	13%
Zinc	11%
Vitamin B6	11%
Protein	10%

Notes
Typical serving is ½ Cup Cooked, 1/7 Cup Dry

62. Brussel Sprouts

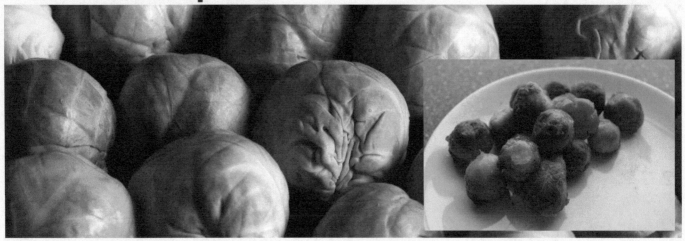

What is Brussel Sprouts?

Brussels sprouts are cruciferous vegetables known for their nutritional density and potential health benefits. They are an excellent source of vitamin K, which plays a crucial role in blood clotting and bone health. Adequate vitamin K intake supports the synthesis of proteins essential for maintaining healthy bones and preventing excessive bleeding.

These vegetables also provide a significant amount of vitamin C, a potent antioxidant that supports the immune system, aids in collagen synthesis for skin health, and helps protect cells from oxidative stress. Brussels sprouts are low in calories and high in fiber, promoting digestive health, regulating blood sugar levels, and contributing to a feeling of fullness.

Incorporating Brussels sprouts into your diet offers a flavorful way to obtain essential vitamins and antioxidants, supporting overall well-being and providing a nutrient-rich addition to a balanced diet.

Top Diseases/Conditions

Brussel Sprouts are identified as a top food for 23 of the Top 100 Diseases and Conditions. Of those, 3 of them rank it between #2 and #10 (Silver Bullets).

3 Silver Bullets	Definition: Top 10 food for each given condition (but not #1)
Cancer: Non-Hodgkin's Lymphoma	Hemorrhoids
Cancer: Prostate	

Nutrients?

One serving (88g, 38 Calories) contains:

9 Significant Nutrients	
Nutrient	DRI Per Serving (Daily Recommended Intake)
Vitamin K	130%
Vitamin C	83%
Vitamin A	22%
Vitamin B6	15%
Iron	15%
Vitamin B9 (Folate)	13%
Manganese	13%
Copper	11%
Potassium	10%

63. Pears

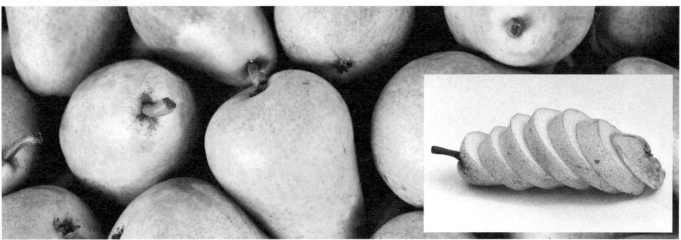

What are Pears?

Pears are sweet and juicy fruits that offer a range of health benefits, making them a delicious and nutritious addition to a balanced diet. These fruits are rich in dietary fiber, promoting digestive health, preventing constipation, and aiding in weight management by providing a sense of fullness.

Pears also contain vitamins and minerals, including vitamin C, which supports immune function and acts as an antioxidant to combat oxidative stress. The presence of potassium in pears contributes to heart health by helping regulate blood pressure.

With a low calorie content, pears make a satisfying and wholesome snack. The natural sugars in pears provide a sweet taste without the need for added sugars. Including pears in your diet offers a tasty way to obtain essential nutrients, contributing to overall well-being and supporting a healthy lifestyle.

Top Diseases/Conditions

Pears are identified as a top food for 9 of the Top 100 Diseases and Conditions. Of those, 1 Diseases and Conditions rank it as #1 (Golden Bullets), while 5 of them rank it between #2 and #10 (Silver Bullets).

1 Golden Bullet	Definition: #1 Top Food for each given condition (other than Water)
Constipation	

5 Silver Bullets	Definition: Top 10 food for each given condition (but not #1)
Aortic Aneurysm	Genital Herpes
Cold Sores	Inguinal Hernia
Diverticulitis	

Nutrients?

One serving (166g, 96 Calories) contains:

2 Significant Nutrients	
Nutrient	DRI Per Serving (Daily Recommended Intake)
Fiber	13%
Copper	11%

64. Beets

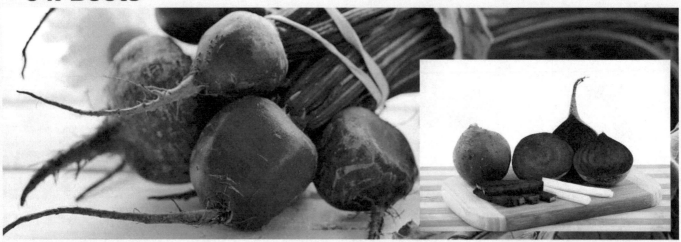

What are Beets?

Beets, vibrant root vegetables, are nutrient-dense and offer numerous health benefits. They are an excellent source of folate, a B-vitamin crucial for DNA synthesis and cell division, making beets beneficial during pregnancy and for overall cellular health.

Rich in manganese, beets support bone health, metabolism, and antioxidant defenses. The iron content contributes to the formation of red blood cells and helps prevent iron deficiency anemia.

Beets are a good source of potassium, supporting heart health by helping regulate blood pressure and fluid balance. Additionally, they contain dietary fiber, promoting digestive health and aiding in weight management.

The natural pigments in beets, like betalains, possess antioxidant and anti-inflammatory properties. Consuming beets may contribute to overall well-being, offering a colorful and flavorful addition to a balanced diet with a diverse range of essential vitamins and minerals.

Top Diseases/Conditions

Beets are identified as a top food for 16 of the Top 100 Diseases and Conditions. Of those, 1 Diseases and Conditions rank it as #1 (Golden Bullets), while 1 of them rank it between #2 and #10 (Silver Bullets).

1 Golden Bullet	Definition: #1 Top Food for each given condition (other than Water)
Chronic Liver Disease/Cirrhosis	

1 Silver Bullet	Definition: Top 10 food for each given condition (but not #1)
Atopic Dermatitis / Eczema	

Nutrients?

One serving (283g, 122 Calories) contains:

12 Significant Nutrients	
Nutrient	DRI Per Serving (Daily Recommended Intake)
Vitamin B9 (Folate)	77%
Manganese	36%
Iron	29%
Potassium	27%
Copper	23%
Fiber	21%
Phosphorus	16%
Vitamin B6	16%
Vitamin B2 (Riboflavin)	16%
Magnesium	16%
Vitamin C	15%
Sodium	15%

65. Cauliflower

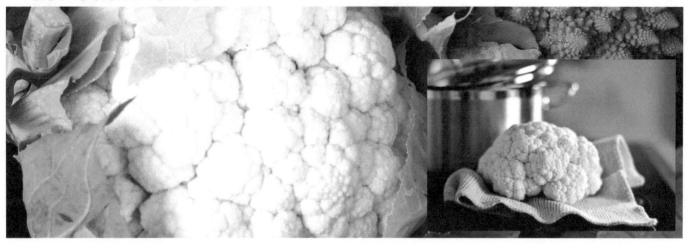

What is Cauliflower?

Cauliflower is a versatile cruciferous vegetable known for its mild flavor and nutrient density. It is an excellent source of vitamin C, a powerful antioxidant that supports the immune system, aids in collagen synthesis for skin health, and protects cells from oxidative stress.

Low in calories and carbohydrates, cauliflower is a great option for those seeking a nutritious, low-calorie vegetable to include in their diet. It also provides fiber, promoting digestive health, regulating blood sugar levels, and aiding in weight management.

Cauliflower's versatility allows it to be used in various dishes, from cauliflower rice to pizza crust alternatives, offering a nutritious substitute for higher-calorie options. Its nutrient profile, including vitamins, minerals, and antioxidants, makes cauliflower a healthy choice for those looking to enhance their overall well-being through a diverse and balanced diet.

Top Diseases/Conditions

Cauliflower is identified as a top food for 19 of the Top 100 Diseases and Conditions. Of those, 1 Diseases and Conditions rank it as #1 (Golden Bullets), while 3 of them rank it between #2 and #10 (Silver Bullets).

1 Golden Bullet	Definition: #1 Top Food for each given condition (other than Water)
Cancer: Bladder	

3 Silver Bullets	Definition: Top 10 food for each given condition (but not #1)
Brain Tumors	Cancer: Prostate
Cancer: Non-Hodgkin's Lymphoma	

Nutrients?

One serving (99g, 25 Calories) contains:

5 Significant Nutrients	
Nutrient	DRI Per Serving (Daily Recommended Intake)
Vitamin C	51%
Vitamin B6	17%
Vitamin B9 (Folate)	14%
Vitamin K	13%
Vitamin B5 (Pantothenic Acid)	13%

66. Pistachios

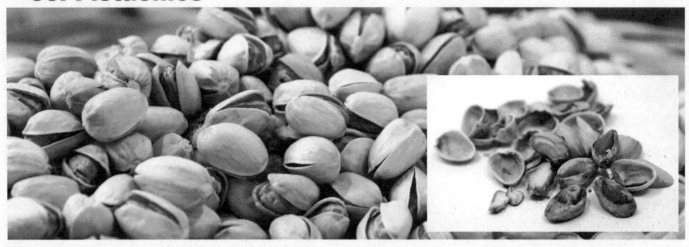

What are Pistachios?

Pistachios are nutrient-rich nuts that offer a host of health benefits. They are an excellent source of copper, a mineral essential for the formation of red blood cells, collagen production, and overall metabolic function. Vitamin B6 in pistachios plays a crucial role in brain development, immune function, and the synthesis of neurotransmitters.

Pistachios contain healthy monounsaturated and polyunsaturated fats, including omega-6 fatty acids, which support heart health by reducing LDL cholesterol levels. These nuts are also rich in antioxidants, such as lutein and zeaxanthin, promoting eye health.

With a satisfying blend of protein and fiber, pistachios contribute to a sense of fullness, making them a beneficial snack for weight management. Incorporating pistachios into a balanced diet provides a tasty and nutritious way to enjoy a range of essential nutrients, supporting overall well-being.

Top Diseases/Conditions

Pistachios are identified as a top food for 5 of the Top 100 Diseases and Conditions. Of those, 1 Diseases and Conditions rank it as #1 (Golden Bullets).

1 Golden Bullet	Definition: #1 Top Food for each given condition (other than Water)
Hypertension	

Nutrients?

One serving (28g, 157 Calories) contains:

9 Significant Nutrients	
Nutrient	DRI Per Serving (Daily Recommended Intake)
Copper	44%
Vitamin B6	38%
"Good" Fat	23%
Omega 6 LA	22%
Phosphorus	20%
Vitamin B1 (Thiamine)	17%
Iron	15%
Manganese	13%
Protein	10%

67. Kefir

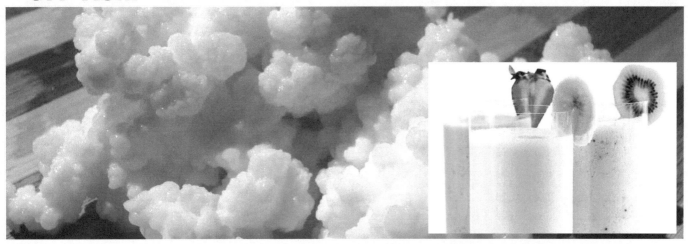

What is Kefir?

Kefir is a fermented dairy product, rich in beneficial nutrients and probiotics that promote digestive health. It contains vitamin B2 (riboflavin), supporting energy metabolism, and aiding in the maintenance of healthy skin, eyes, and nerve functions. Kefir is also a good source of phosphorus and calcium, essential minerals for bone health, teeth, and overall cellular function.

One of the key health benefits of kefir lies in its probiotic content. Probiotics are live microorganisms that confer various health advantages, including improved gut health, enhanced immune function, and the potential alleviation of digestive issues. The fermentation process of kefir enhances its digestibility and nutrient absorption.

Incorporating kefir into your diet provides a delicious and versatile way to enjoy the nutritional benefits of probiotics, vitamins, and minerals, contributing to a balanced and gut-friendly approach to overall well-being.

Top Diseases/Conditions

Kefir is identified as a top food for 10 of the Top 100 Diseases and Conditions. Of those, 4 of them rank it between #2 and #10 (Silver Bullets).

4 Silver Bullets	Definition: Top 10 food for each given condition (but not #1)
Atopic Dermatitis / Eczema	Contact Dermatitis
Autism	Urinary Tract Infection

Nutrients?

One serving (244g, 139 Calories) contains:

7 Significant Nutrients	
Nutrient	DRI Per Serving (Daily Recommended Intake)
Vitamin B2 (Riboflavin)	38%
Phosphorus	33%
Calcium	30%
Protein	14%
Vitamin B12	13%
Potassium	11%
Zinc	10%

68. Tuna

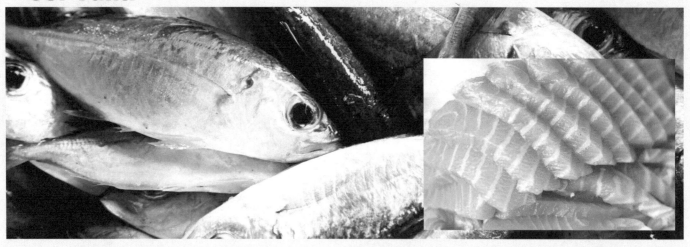

What is Tuna?

Tuna is a nutrient-rich fish that offers a variety of health benefits. It is an excellent source of omega-3 fatty acids, specifically DHA (docosahexaenoic acid) and EPA (eicosapentaenoic acid), which support heart health, brain function, and contribute to anti-inflammatory effects in the body. These fatty acids are crucial for cognitive development and may help reduce the risk of cardiovascular diseases.

Tuna also provides selenium, a trace mineral with antioxidant properties that support immune function and thyroid health. Vitamin B12 in tuna is essential for energy metabolism, nervous system function, and the formation of red blood cells. Additionally, tuna is a high-quality protein source, promoting muscle development and repair.

Incorporating tuna into a balanced diet offers a convenient and delicious way to obtain these essential nutrients, contributing to overall well-being and supporting various aspects of health.

Top Diseases/Conditions

Tuna is identified as a top food for 14 of the Top 100 Diseases and Conditions. Of those, 1 Diseases and Conditions rank it as #1 (Golden Bullets), while 3 of them rank it between #2 and #10 (Silver Bullets).

1 Golden Bullet	Definition: #1 Top Food for each given condition (other than Water)
Fibromyalgia	

3 Silver Bullet	Definition: Top 10 food for each given condition (but not #1)
Cancer: Thyroid	Parkinsons
Hypothyroidism	

Nutrients?

One serving (85g, 109 Calories) contains:

10 Significant Nutrients	
Nutrient	DRI Per Serving (Daily Recommended Intake)
Omega-3 DHA	214%
Selenium	101%
Omega-3 EPA	79%
Vitamin B12	42%
Protein	36%
Vitamin B3 (Niacin)	31%
Phosphorus	26%
Sodium	21%
Vitamin B6	15%
Iron	10%

69. Peas

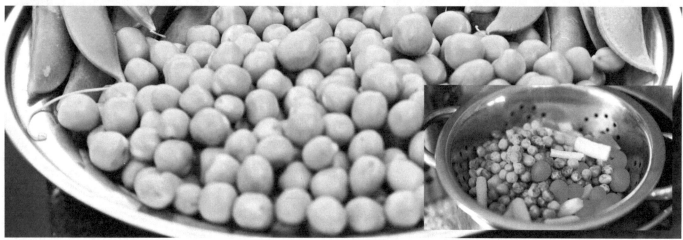

What are Peas?

Peas are nutrient-packed legumes that contribute to a well-rounded and nutritious diet. They are rich in vitamin C, an antioxidant that supports immune function, skin health, and aids in collagen synthesis. Vitamin A in peas promotes vision, immune function, and skin integrity.

Thiamine (vitamin B1) in peas plays a key role in energy metabolism, ensuring proper utilization of carbohydrates for energy. Copper, another essential mineral found in peas, supports the formation of red blood cells and assists in maintaining a healthy immune system.

Peas are an excellent source of vitamin K, vital for blood clotting and bone health. The combination of vitamins, minerals, and dietary fiber in peas makes them a healthy choice for promoting digestive health, supporting a strong immune system, and contributing to overall well-being. Their versatility and nutritional profile make peas a valuable addition to a balanced and varied diet.

Top Diseases/Conditions

Peas are identified as a top food for 21 of the Top 100 Diseases and Conditions. Of those, 1 Diseases and Conditions rank it as #1 (Golden Bullets).

1 Golden Bullet	Definition: #1 Top Food for each given condition (other than Water)
Inguinal Hernia	

Nutrients?

One serving (145g, 117 Calories) contains:

17 Significant Nutrients	
Nutrient	DRI Per Serving (Daily Recommended Intake)
Vitamin C	64%
Vitamin A	37%
Vitamin B1 (Thiamine)	33%
Copper	33%
Vitamin K	30%
Iron	26%
Manganese	26%
Vitamin B9 (Folate)	24%
Phosphorus	22%
Fiber	19%
Vitamin B3 (Niacin)	19%
Zinc	16%
Vitamin B6	15%
Vitamin B2 (Riboflavin)	15%
Protein	14%
Magnesium	11%
Potassium	10%

70. Prunes

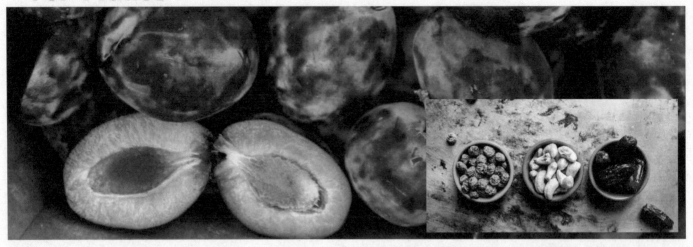

What are Prunes?

Prunes are dried plums known for their sweet and distinctive flavor, and they offer a range of health benefits. Rich in vitamin K, prunes contribute to blood clotting and bone health, playing a crucial role in maintaining skeletal integrity. This vitamin is particularly important for supporting healthy bone density and reducing the risk of fractures.

The drying process concentrates the nutritional content of prunes, providing a concentrated source of fiber, vitamins, and minerals. Prunes are well-regarded for their natural laxative effect, promoting digestive regularity and potentially preventing constipation.

Additionally, prunes contain antioxidants that combat oxidative stress, supporting overall cellular health. Incorporating prunes into a balanced diet offers a delicious and convenient way to enjoy their nutritional benefits, making them a nutrient-dense snack that contributes to both digestive and bone health.

Top Diseases/Conditions

Prunes are identified as a top food for 7 of the Top 100 Diseases and Conditions. Of those, 1 Diseases and Conditions rank it as #1 (Golden Bullets).

1 Golden Bullet	Definition: #1 Top Food for each given condition (other than Water)
Constipation	

Nutrients?

One serving (30g, 95 Calories) contains:

3 Significant Nutrients	
Nutrient	DRI Per Serving (Daily Recommended Intake)
Vitamin K	20%
Copper	13%
Vitamin A	10%

71. Kiwi

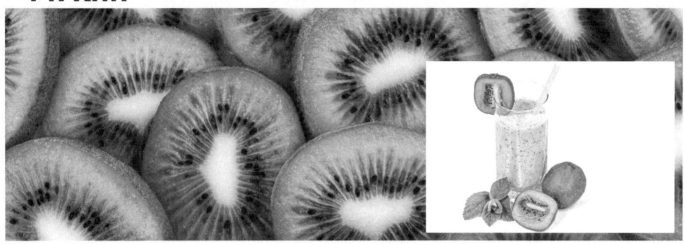

What are Kiwis?

Kiwis, also known as kiwifruits, are small, vibrant green fruits that pack a nutritional punch. They are an excellent source of vitamin C, providing more than the recommended daily intake in a single serving. Vitamin C supports immune function, collagen synthesis, and acts as a potent antioxidant, protecting cells from oxidative stress.

Kiwi fruits also contain vitamin K, essential for blood clotting and bone health. Adequate vitamin K intake contributes to maintaining strong and healthy bones.

These fruits are rich in dietary fiber, aiding digestion and promoting a feeling of fullness. Additionally, kiwis contain a range of antioxidants, including flavonoids and carotenoids, which contribute to overall health by combating inflammation and oxidative damage.

Incorporating kiwis into a balanced diet offers a tasty and nutritious way to enhance immune function, support bone health, and enjoy the benefits of a variety of essential nutrients.

Top Diseases/Conditions

Kiwis are identified as a top food for 8 of the Top 100 Diseases and Conditions. However, they were not identified as a Top 10 food for any of those Top 100 Diseases and conditions.

Nutrients?

One serving (148g, 90 Calories) contains:

6 Significant Nutrients	
Nutrient	DRI Per Serving *(Daily Recommended Intake)*
Vitamin C	152%
Vitamin K	50%
Copper	22%
Vitamin E	15%
Potassium	14%
Fiber	12%

72. Coconut Oil

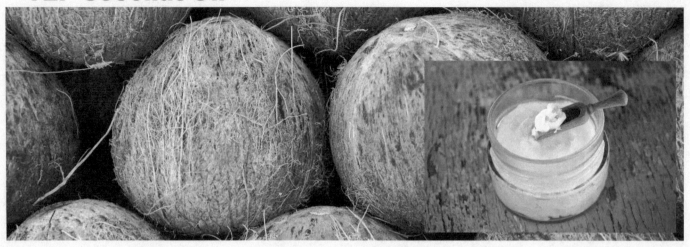

What is Coconut Oil?

Coconut oil is a versatile cooking oil derived from the flesh of mature coconuts. It is predominantly composed of saturated fats, including medium-chain triglycerides (MCTs). While high in saturated fats, the unique fatty acid profile of MCTs in coconut oil may offer certain health benefits. MCTs are quickly absorbed and converted into energy, making them a potential source of quick fuel for the body.

Some studies suggest that the MCTs in coconut oil may aid in weight management, support heart health by raising HDL (good) cholesterol, and possess antimicrobial properties. Coconut oil is also heat-stable, making it suitable for cooking at higher temperatures.

However, moderation is key, as excessive consumption of saturated fats may have adverse effects on cardiovascular health. It's recommended to incorporate coconut oil into a balanced diet to enjoy its potential benefits while considering overall dietary fat intake.

Top Diseases/Conditions

Coconut Oil is identified as a top food for 9 of the Top 100 Diseases and Conditions. However, they were not identified as a Top 10 food for any of those Top 100 Diseases and conditions.

Nutrients?

One serving (13g, 116 Calories) contains:

1 Significant Nutrient	
Nutrient	DRI Per Serving (Daily Recommended Intake)
"Good" Fat	20%

73. Grapes

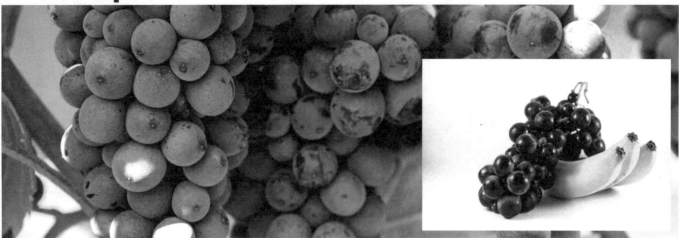

What are Grapes?

Grapes are delicious and nutritious fruits known for their natural sweetness and a variety of health benefits. They are rich in copper, a trace mineral that plays a role in the formation of red blood cells and connective tissues. Copper also acts as an antioxidant, contributing to the body's defense against oxidative stress.

Vitamin K, found in grapes, is essential for blood clotting and bone health. Adequate vitamin K intake supports proper calcium utilization and bone mineralization.

Furthermore, grapes provide a notable dose of vitamin C, a potent antioxidant vital for immune function, collagen synthesis, and skin health. The antioxidants in grapes, including resveratrol, may contribute to cardiovascular health by promoting healthy blood vessels.

Incorporating grapes into a balanced diet adds natural sweetness while offering a spectrum of nutrients that contribute to overall well-being.

Top Diseases/Conditions

Grapes are identified as a top food for 9 of the Top 100 Diseases and Conditions. Of those, 1 Diseases and Conditions rank it as #1 (Golden Bullets).

1 Golden Bullet	Definition: #1 Top Food for each given condition (other than Water)
Peptic Ulcer	

Nutrients?

One serving (126g, 87 Calories) contains:

3 Significant Nutrients	
Nutrient	DRI Per Serving (Daily Recommended Intake)
Copper	22%
Vitamin K	15%
Vitamin C	15%

74. Lettuce

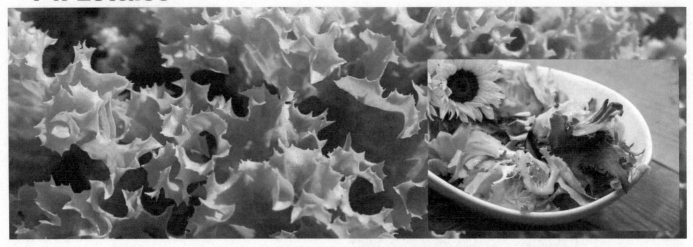

What is Lettuce?

Lettuce, a leafy green vegetable, is a low-calorie, nutrient-rich addition to a healthy diet. It is particularly abundant in vitamin K, a crucial nutrient for blood clotting and bone health. Adequate vitamin K intake supports the body's ability to form blood clots and contributes to maintaining strong and healthy bones.

Lettuce also provides a notable amount of vitamin A, important for vision, immune function, and skin health. Vitamin A is a powerful antioxidant that plays a role in maintaining the health of various tissues in the body.

The high water content in lettuce makes it hydrating and a good choice for promoting overall hydration. Incorporating lettuce into salads and sandwiches is an excellent way to increase fiber intake and add essential vitamins to support overall well-being and a healthy lifestyle.

Top Diseases/Conditions

Lettuce is identified as a top food for 5 of the Top 100 Diseases and Conditions. However, they were not identified as a Top 10 food for any of those Top 100 Diseases and conditions.

Nutrients?

One serving (89g, 13 Calories) contains:

| 2 Significant Nutrients ||
Nutrient	DRI Per Serving (Daily Recommended Intake)
Vitamin K	18%
Vitamin A	15%

75. Apple Cider Vinegar

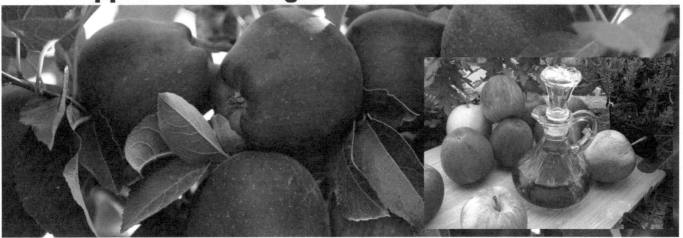

What is Apple Cider Vinegar?

Apple Cider Vinegar (ACV) is a fermented liquid made from crushed apples. It contains acetic acid, which is believed to contribute to its potential health benefits. ACV has been associated with various positive effects, including improved digestion and blood sugar control.

The acetic acid in ACV may aid digestion by promoting the growth of beneficial bacteria in the gut. Some studies suggest that it may help lower blood sugar levels after meals, offering potential benefits for individuals with insulin resistance or diabetes.

Additionally, ACV has been linked to weight loss by increasing feelings of fullness and reducing calorie intake.

It's important to note that while ACV has potential health benefits, excessive consumption may lead to negative effects, and it should be used in moderation. Incorporating small amounts of ACV into your diet, such as in salad dressings or diluted with water, can be a flavorful and potentially health-promoting addition.

Top Diseases/Conditions

Apple Cider Vinegar is identified as a top food for 5 of the Top 100 Diseases and Conditions. However, they were not identified as a Top 10 food for any of those Top 100 Diseases and conditions.

Nutrients?

One serving (14g, 3 Calories) contains no nutrients that are at least 10% DRI.

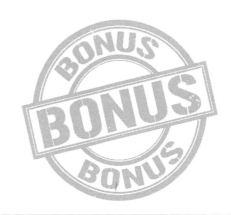

Top 10 Foods with Most Golden Bullets		
	Food	Golden Bullets
1	Water	100
2	Salmon	40
3	Spinach	22
4	Mackeral	20
5	Broccoli	15
6	Kale	15
7	Almonds	14
8	Herring	14
9	Blueberries	10
10	Oranges	10

76. Green Beans

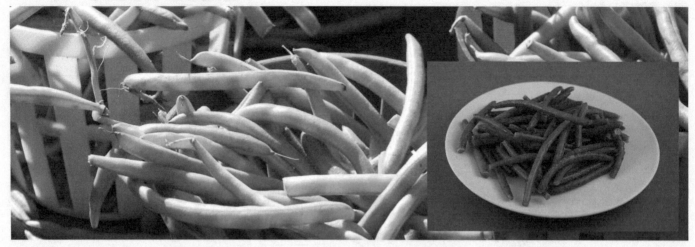

What are Green Beans?

Green Beans, also known as string beans or snap beans, are nutritious vegetables with various health benefits. They are rich in thiamine, a B-vitamin essential for energy metabolism and maintaining proper nerve function. Thiamine helps convert carbohydrates into energy, supporting overall vitality.

Green beans are a low-calorie food packed with fiber, vitamins, and minerals. The fiber content aids in digestion, promotes a feeling of fullness, and supports a healthy digestive system.

These beans also provide essential nutrients like vitamin C, vitamin K, and folate. Vitamin C acts as an antioxidant, supporting the immune system and collagen production, while vitamin K is crucial for blood clotting and bone health. Folate is important for cell division and the formation of DNA.

Incorporating green beans into a balanced diet contributes to overall well-being, providing valuable nutrients that support energy production and various bodily functions.

Top Diseases/Conditions

Green Beans are identified as a top food for 15 of the Top 100 Diseases and Conditions. However, they were not identified as a Top 10 food for any of those Top 100 Diseases and conditions.

Nutrients?

One serving (83g, 26 Calories) contains:

5 Significant Nutrients	
Nutrient	DRI Per Serving (Daily Recommended Intake)
Vitamin B1 (Thiamine)	101%
Vitamin A	19%
Vitamin C	15%
Iron	10%
Vitamin K	10%

77. Cranberries

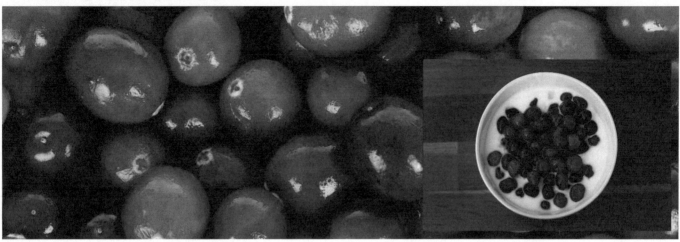

What are Cranberries?

Cranberries are vibrant red berries known for their tart flavor and numerous health benefits. They are rich in manganese, a trace mineral that plays a role in bone formation, blood clotting, and reducing inflammation. Manganese also contributes to energy metabolism, supporting the body's utilization of nutrients for energy.

Cranberries are an excellent source of vitamin C, a powerful antioxidant essential for immune function, collagen synthesis, and skin health. The antioxidant properties of vitamin C help protect cells from oxidative stress and support overall well-being.

These berries are also associated with urinary tract health, as certain compounds in cranberries may help prevent urinary tract infections by inhibiting the adherence of bacteria to the urinary tract lining.

Incorporating cranberries into a balanced diet, whether fresh, dried, or in juice form, adds a burst of flavor and provides essential nutrients that contribute to overall health and vitality.

Top Diseases/Conditions

Cranberries are identified as a top food for 7 of the Top 100 Diseases and Conditions. Of those, 2 Diseases and Conditions rank it as #1 (Golden Bullets).

2 Golden Bullets	Definition: #1 Top Food for each given condition (other than Water)
Chronic Kidney Disease	Urinary Tract Infection

Nutrients?

One serving (140g, 64 Calories) contains:

6 Significant Nutrients	
Nutrient	DRI Per Serving (Daily Recommended Intake)
Manganese	22%
Vitamin C	21%
Fiber	17%
Copper	14%
Vitamin E	11%
Vitamin B6	10%

78. Sunflower Seeds

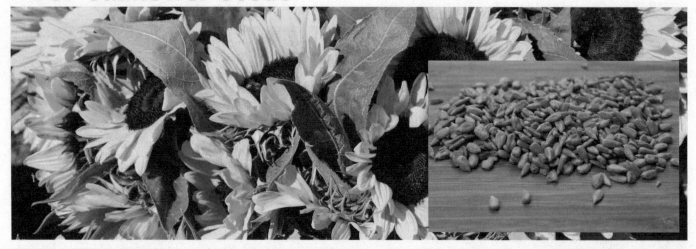

What are Sunflower Seeds?

Sunflower seeds (healthfully eaten as kernals) are nutrient-packed kernels derived from the sunflower plant. These seeds are a rich source of various essential nutrients. They contain vitamin E, a potent antioxidant that helps protect cells from oxidative damage and supports skin health. Copper, another mineral found in sunflower seeds, plays a role in the formation of red blood cells and connective tissues.

Sunflower seeds are a significant source of omega-6 fatty acids, which contribute to heart health and may help reduce inflammation in the body. Additionally, these seeds provide thiamine (vitamin B1) and vitamin B6, both crucial for energy metabolism and the proper functioning of the nervous system.

Incorporating sunflower seeds into your diet offers a convenient and tasty way to access these nutrients, promoting overall well-being and supporting various bodily functions. Enjoy them as a snack, sprinkle them on salads, or use them in recipes to enhance the nutritional content of your meals.

Top Diseases/Conditions

Sunflower Seeds are identified as a top food for 8 of the Top 100 Diseases and Conditions. Of those, 1

Diseases and Conditions rank it as #1 (Golden Bullets), while 1 of them rank it between #2 and #10 (Silver Bullets).

1 Golden Bullet	Definition: #1 Top Food for each given condition (other than Water)
Hypertension	

1 Silver Bullet	Definition: Top 10 food for each given condition (but not #1)
Asthma	

Nutrients?

One serving (Kernals, 28g, 164 Calories) contains:

15 Significant Nutrients	
Nutrient	DRI Per Serving (Daily Recommended Intake)
Vitamin E	62%
Copper	56%
Omega 6 LA	38%
Vitamin B1 (Thiamine)	33%
Vitamin B6	31%
Selenium	27%
"Good" Fat	27%
Phosphorus	26%
Manganese	22%
Magnesium	22%
Iron	19%
Vitamin B9 (Folate)	16%
Vitamin B3 (Niacin)	14%
Zinc	13%
Protein	10%

79. Chamomile Tea

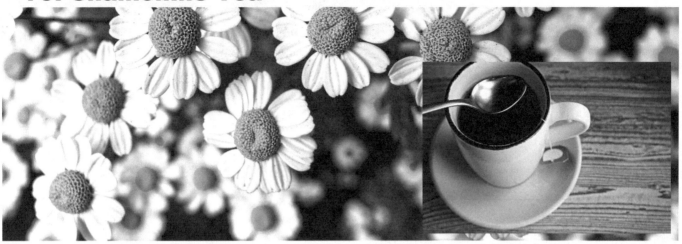

What is Chamomile Tea?

Chamomile tea is an herbal infusion made from the dried flowers of the chamomile plant, scientifically known as Matricaria chamomilla or Chamaemelum nobile. This caffeine-free tea has been consumed for centuries and is renowned for its potential health benefits.

Chamomile tea is prized for its calming properties, often used to promote relaxation and alleviate stress. It contains antioxidants, such as apigenin, which may have anti-inflammatory effects and contribute to overall well-being. The tea is also commonly enjoyed for its potential to aid in digestion, alleviate insomnia, and soothe mild discomfort.

Furthermore, chamomile tea is known for its mild, floral flavor, making it a popular choice for those seeking a comforting and soothing beverage. Whether sipped before bedtime or as a gentle remedy for stress, chamomile tea offers a natural and delightful way to relax and support various aspects of health.

Top Diseases/Conditions

Chamomile Tea is identified as a top food for 5 of the Top 100 Diseases and Conditions. Of those, 1 Diseases and Conditions rank it as #1 (Golden Bullets), while 1 of them rank it between #2 and #10 (Silver Bullets).

1 Golden Bullet	Definition: #1 Top Food for each given condition (other than Water)
Insomnia	

1 Silver Bullet	Definition: Top 10 food for each given condition (but not #1)
Streptococcal Pharyngitis	

Nutrients?

One serving (227g, 2 Calories) contains no nutrients that are at least 10% DRI.

80. Cucumbers

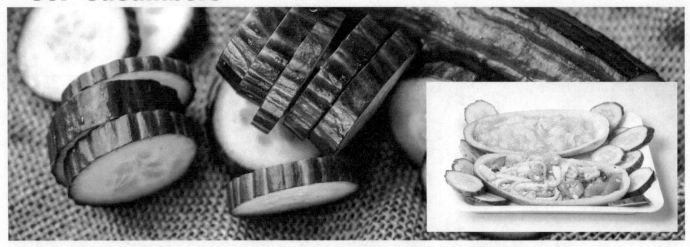

What are Cucumbers?

Cucumbers are crisp, refreshing vegetables belonging to the gourd family, known for their hydrating and nutritious qualities. They are an excellent source of vitamin K, a fat-soluble vitamin essential for blood clotting and bone health. Adequate vitamin K intake supports proper calcium utilization, contributing to bone strength and density.

Beyond their vitamin K content, cucumbers are low in calories and provide hydration due to their high water content, making them a hydrating snack. They also offer a variety of antioxidants, including flavonoids and tannins, which may have anti-inflammatory and anti-cancer properties.

Cucumbers are a versatile addition to salads, sandwiches, or enjoyed on their own as a crunchy snack. Their hydrating nature, coupled with essential nutrients like vitamin K, makes cucumbers a nutritious choice for supporting overall health and well-being.

Top Diseases/Conditions

Cucumbers are identified as a top food for 5 of the Top 100 Diseases and Conditions. However, they were not identified as a Top 10 food for any of those Top 100 Diseases and conditions.

Nutrients?

One serving (99g, 15 Calories) contains:

1 Significant Nutrient	
Nutrient	DRI Per Serving (Daily Recommended Intake)
Vitamin K	14%

144

81. Celery

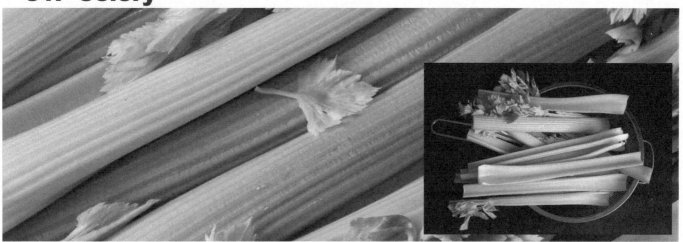

What is Celery?

Celery is a crisp and crunchy vegetable with a wealth of health benefits. It contains vitamin K, an essential nutrient for blood clotting and bone health, contributing to the maintenance of strong and healthy bones. Additionally, celery provides vitamin A, which is crucial for vision, immune function, and skin health.

Rich in folate, celery plays a role in DNA synthesis and cell division, supporting overall cellular function and growth. Celery is also low in calories and high in water content, making it a hydrating and nutritious snack. Its natural fibers contribute to digestive health by aiding in regular bowel movements.

Furthermore, celery is known for its potential anti-inflammatory properties and is often recommended as part of a balanced diet for those looking to manage blood pressure and support heart health. Incorporating celery into salads, soups, or enjoying it as a crunchy snack provides a tasty and healthful addition to a well-rounded diet.

Top Diseases/Conditions

Celery is identified as a top food for 7 of the Top 100 Diseases and Conditions. However, they were not identified as a Top 10 food for any of those Top 100 Diseases and conditions.

Nutrients?

One serving (110g, 18 Calories) contains:

| 3 Significant Nutrients ||
Nutrient	DRI Per Serving (Daily Recommended Intake)
Vitamin K	27%
Vitamin A	16%
Vitamin B9 (Folate)	10%

82. Peanuts

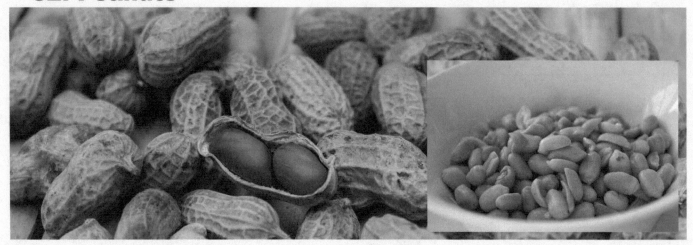

What are Peanuts?

Peanuts, although commonly mistaken for nuts, are actually legumes and boast a variety of health benefits. They are a rich source of copper, a trace mineral essential for the formation of red blood cells and overall immune system function. Additionally, peanuts contain omega-6 fatty acids, contributing to heart health and supporting normal growth and development.

Manganese, another mineral found in peanuts, plays a crucial role in bone formation, blood clotting, and reducing inflammation. Peanuts are also a good source of niacin (vitamin B3), important for energy metabolism and the maintenance of healthy skin.

Including peanuts in your diet provides a satisfying and nutrient-dense snack. However, moderation is key due to their calorie density. Choose unsalted and dry-roasted peanuts to maximize health benefits while minimizing added salt and oil. The combination of essential nutrients in peanuts makes them a tasty and nutritious addition to a well-balanced diet.

Top Diseases/Conditions

Peanuts are identified as a top food for 3 of the Top 100 Diseases and Conditions. Of those, 1 of them rank it between #2 and #10 (Silver Bullets).

1 Silver Bullet	Definition: Top 10 food for each given condition (but not #1)
Premenstrual Syndrome	

Nutrients?

One serving (28g, 159 Calories) contains:

13 Significant Nutrients	
Nutrient	DRI Per Serving *(Daily Recommended Intake)*
Copper	33%
Omega 6 LA	26%
"Good" Fat	25%
Manganese	22%
Vitamin B3 (Niacin)	21%
Vitamin B9 (Folate)	17%
Vitamin B1 (Thiamine)	17%
Iron	16%
Vitamin E	15%
Phosphorus	15%
Protein	13%
Magnesium	11%
Vitamin B5 (Pantothenic Acid)	10%

83. Soybeans

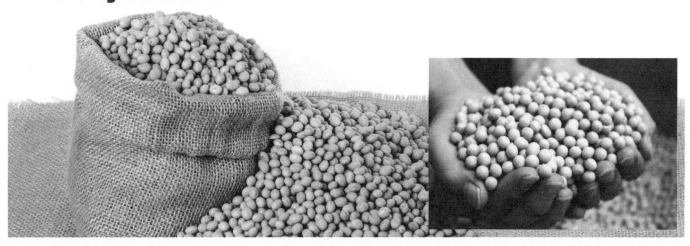

What are Soybeans?

Soybeans, versatile legumes consumed in various forms like edamame, offer a wealth of nutritional benefits. Rich in iron, soybeans contribute to the formation of red blood cells, aiding in the prevention of anemia. Copper, another essential mineral in soybeans, plays a role in maintaining healthy connective tissues and supporting the immune system.

Soybeans are a source of omega-3 alpha-linolenic acid (ALA), promoting heart health by reducing inflammation and supporting optimal cardiovascular function. Manganese in soybeans contributes to bone formation, blood clotting, and overall antioxidant defenses.

Additionally, soybeans are packed with phosphorus, crucial for bone health and energy metabolism. As a complete protein source, soybeans provide all essential amino acids, making them an excellent plant-based protein option for vegetarians and vegans.

Incorporating soybeans into your diet, whether as edamame, tofu, or soy milk, offers a nutrient-dense and plant-based protein alternative with diverse health benefits, supporting overall well-being.

Top Diseases/Conditions

Soybeans are identified as a top food for 19 of the Top 100 Diseases and Conditions. Of those, 1 Diseases and Conditions rank it as #1 (Golden Bullets), while 1 of them rank it between #2 and #10 (Silver Bullets).

1 Golden Bullet	Definition: #1 Top Food for each given condition (other than Water)
Inflammatory Bowel Disease	

1 Silver Bullet	Definition: Top 10 food for each given condition (but not #1)
Iron Deficiency Anemia	

Nutrients?

One serving (128g, 222 Calories) contains:

20 Significant Nutrients	
Nutrient	DRI Per Serving *(Daily Recommended Intake)*
Iron	82%
Copper	58%
Omega-3 ALA	48%
Manganese	45%
Phosphorus	45%
Protein	38%
Omega 6 LA	34%
Vitamin B2 (Riboflavin)	29%
Magnesium	26%
Vitamin B6	23%
Vitamin K	20%
Fiber	20%
Potassium	19%
Vitamin B1 (Thiamine)	19%
Vitamin B9 (Folate)	17%
Selenium	17%
Zinc	14%
Calcium	13%
"Good" Fat	13%
Choline	11%

84. Mustard Greens

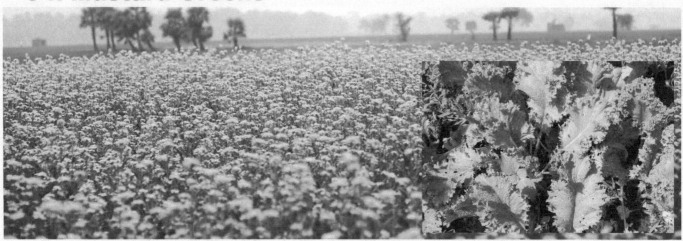

What are Mustard Greens?

Mustard greens are leafy vegetables known for their robust flavor and numerous health benefits. Packed with vitamin K, these greens play a crucial role in blood clotting and bone health. Adequate vitamin K intake supports overall cardiovascular health and helps maintain strong and healthy bones.

Rich in vitamin A, mustard greens contribute to vision health, immune system function, and the maintenance of skin and mucous membranes. The beta-carotene in vitamin A acts as a powerful antioxidant, protecting cells from damage.

Mustard greens are low in calories and high in fiber, promoting digestive health and helping with weight management. They also contain essential minerals like calcium and iron, further supporting bone health and preventing anemia.

Incorporating mustard greens into your diet, whether raw in salads, sautéed, or blended into smoothies, provides a tasty and nutrient-packed addition that supports overall wellness.

Top Diseases/Conditions

Mustard Greens are identified as a top food for 4 of the Top 100 Diseases and Conditions. However, they were not identified as a Top 10 food for any of those Top 100 Diseases and conditions.

Nutrients?

One serving (56g, 15 Calories) contains:

7 Significant Nutrients	
Nutrient	DRI Per Serving (Daily Recommended Intake)
Vitamin K	232%
Vitamin A	196%
Vitamin C	44%
Vitamin B9 (Folate)	26%
Manganese	13%
Copper	11%
Iron	10%

85. Asparagus

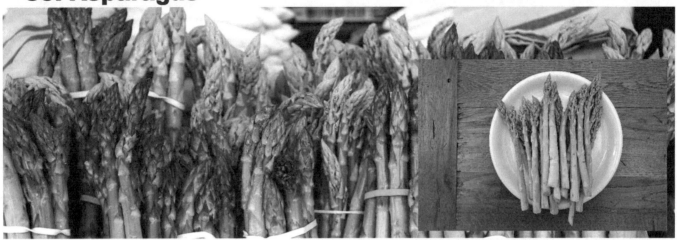

What is Asparagus?

Asparagus, a delicious and nutritious vegetable, offers a variety of health benefits. Rich in vitamin K, asparagus plays a crucial role in blood clotting and bone health, supporting overall cardiovascular and skeletal well-being. Adequate vitamin K intake is essential for optimal bone density and strength.

Additionally, asparagus contains iron, a vital mineral for transporting oxygen in the blood and preventing fatigue and anemia. The presence of vitamin A in asparagus contributes to healthy vision, immune function, and skin integrity. Copper, another mineral found in asparagus, supports the formation of red blood cells and helps maintain proper nerve function.

Low in calories and high in fiber, asparagus promotes digestive health and can contribute to weight management. Including asparagus in your diet provides a tasty and nutrient-dense option that supports various aspects of your overall health.

Top Diseases/Conditions

Asparagus is identified as a top food for 9 of the Top 100 Diseases and Conditions. Of those, 2 of them rank it between #2 and #10 (Silver Bullets).

2 Silver Bullets	Definition: Top 10 food for each given condition (but not #1)
Rosacea	Schizophrenia

Nutrients?

One serving (93g, 19 Calories) contains:

7 Significant Nutrients	
Nutrient	DRI Per Serving (Daily Recommended Intake)
Vitamin K	32%
Iron	25%
Vitamin A	23%
Copper	23%
Vitamin B9 (Folate)	12%
Vitamin B1 (Thiamine)	12%
Vitamin B2 (Riboflavin)	11%

86. Red Wine

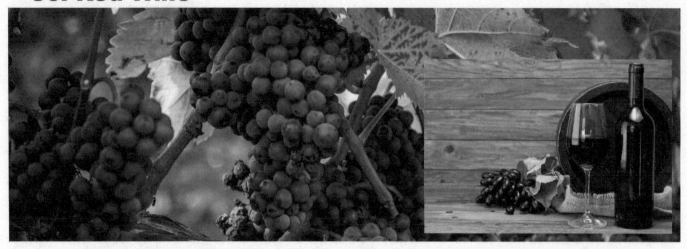

What is Red Wine?

Red Wine, made from fermented dark-colored grapes, offers potential health benefits when consumed in moderation. Rich in antioxidants like resveratrol, red wine may have cardio-protective effects by improving heart health and reducing the risk of coronary artery disease. Resveratrol has been associated with anti-inflammatory and anti-aging properties.

Moderate consumption of red wine has been linked to improvements in cholesterol levels, potentially raising high-density lipoprotein (HDL or "good" cholesterol) while reducing low-density lipoprotein (LDL or "bad" cholesterol) oxidation.

Some studies suggest that the polyphenols in red wine may contribute to cognitive function and lower the risk of neurodegenerative diseases.

It's crucial to emphasize moderation, as excessive alcohol consumption can have adverse health effects.

Top Diseases/Conditions

Red Wine is identified as a top food for 10 of the Top 100 Diseases and Conditions. However, they were not identified as a Top 10 food for any of those Top 100 Diseases and conditions.

Nutrients?

One serving (142g, 122 Calories) contains no nutrients that are at least 10% DRI.

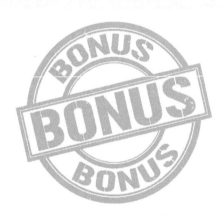

Top 10 Foods with Most Total Bullets (Gold + Silver)		
	Food	Golden Bullets
1	Water	100
2	Salmon	79
3	Spinach	56
4	Mackeral	55
5	Broccoli	51
6	Kale	50
7	Strawberries	40
8	Walnuts	39
9	Herring	37
10	Whole Oats	35

87. Turnip Greens

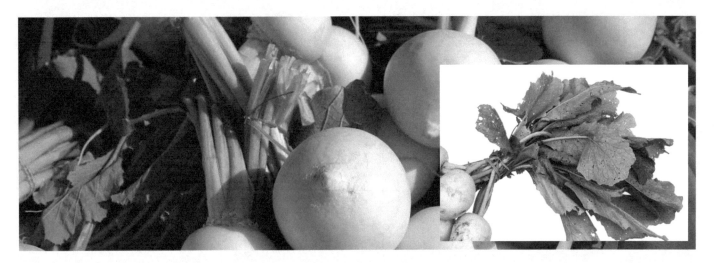

What is Turnip Greens?

Turnip greens, the leafy tops of the turnip plant, are a nutrient-dense leafy green vegetable with several health benefits. Packed with vitamin A, these greens contribute to eye health, immune function, and skin maintenance. Abundant in vitamin K, they play a crucial role in bone health and blood clotting.

Additionally, turnip greens are an excellent source of vitamin C, a powerful antioxidant that supports the immune system and aids in collagen production for skin health.

Rich in fiber, turnip greens promote digestive health by supporting regular bowel movements and providing a sense of fullness. They also contain minerals like calcium and iron, contributing to bone strength and preventing anemia.

Incorporating turnip greens into your diet can be a flavorful and nutritious way to enhance overall well-being, supporting various bodily functions and providing a spectrum of essential vitamins and minerals.

Top Diseases/Conditions

Turnip Greens are identified as a top food for 3 of the Top 100 Diseases and Conditions. Of those, 1 of them rank it between #2 and #10 (Silver Bullets).

1 Silver Bullet	Definition: Top 10 food for each given condition (but not #1)
Osteoporosis	

Nutrients?

One serving (55g, 18 Calories) contains:

8 Significant Nutrients	
Nutrient	DRI Per Serving (Daily Recommended Intake)
Vitamin A	212%
Vitamin K	115%
Vitamin C	37%
Vitamin B9 (Folate)	27%
Copper	22%
Manganese	13%
Vitamin E	11%
Calcium	11%

88. Buckwheat

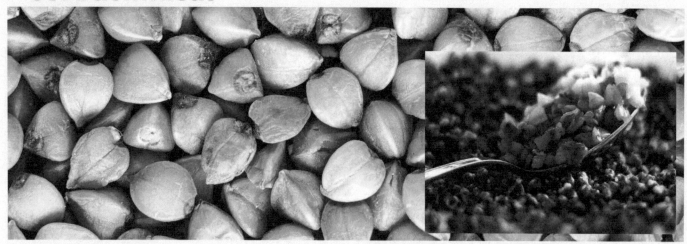

What is Buckwheat?

Buckwheat is a nutrient-rich whole grain that offers a range of health benefits. Packed with manganese, it plays a vital role in bone formation, blood clotting, and reducing inflammation. The presence of iron in buckwheat supports oxygen transport in the blood, preventing anemia and promoting overall energy levels.

Rich in magnesium, buckwheat contributes to muscle and nerve function, blood sugar regulation, and bone health. Its high-fiber content aids in digestion, promoting a healthy gut and contributing to feelings of fullness.

Moreover, buckwheat is gluten-free, making it a suitable option for individuals with gluten sensitivities or celiac disease. It contains antioxidants that combat oxidative stress in the body, potentially reducing the risk of chronic diseases.

Incorporating buckwheat into your diet can be a delicious and versatile way to enhance nutritional intake while reaping the benefits of its essential minerals and fiber.

Top Diseases/Conditions

Buckwheat is identified as a top food for 9 of the Top 100 Diseases and Conditions. Of those, 1 Diseases and Conditions rank it as #1 (Golden Bullets).

1 Golden Bullet	Definition: #1 Top Food for each given condition (other than Water)
Celiac Disease	

Nutrients?

One serving (1/4 Cup Groats Flour, 32g, 107 Calories) contains:

8 Significant Nutrients	
Nutrient	DRI Per Serving (Daily Recommended Intake)
Manganese	28%
Magnesium	19%
Copper	18%
Iron	16%
Phosphorus	15%
Vitamin B6	14%
Vitamin B3 (Niacin)	12%
Vitamin B1 (Thiamine)	11%

Typical serving is ½ Cup Cooked, 1/8 Cup Dry

89. Bok Choy

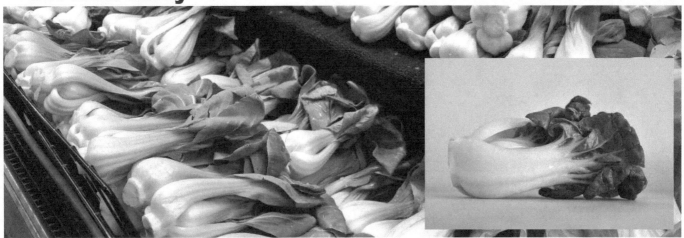

What is Bok Choy?

Bok Choy, a cruciferous vegetable, is a powerhouse of nutrients that contributes to overall health. Rich in vitamin K, bok choy supports blood clotting and bone health, playing a crucial role in maintaining a strong skeletal system. Its high vitamin C content boosts the immune system, promoting the body's ability to fight off infections and supporting skin health.

Additionally, bok choy is low in calories and contains a variety of essential minerals, including calcium, potassium, and manganese. The presence of fiber aids in digestion and contributes to a feeling of fullness, making it a great choice for weight management. As part of the Brassicaceae family, bok choy also contains compounds with potential anti-cancer properties.

Incorporating bok choy into your diet provides a tasty and nutritious way to enhance your overall well-being, supporting various bodily functions and promoting a balanced, healthy lifestyle.

Top Diseases/Conditions

Bok Choy is identified as a top food for 11 of the Top 100 Diseases and Conditions. However, they were not identified as a Top 10 food for any of those Top 100 Diseases and conditions.

Nutrients?

One serving (70g, 9 Calories) contains:

4 Significant Nutrients	
Nutrient	DRI Per Serving (Daily Recommended Intake)
Vitamin A	104%
Vitamin C	35%
Vitamin K	27%
Vitamin B9 (Folate)	12%

90. Mushrooms

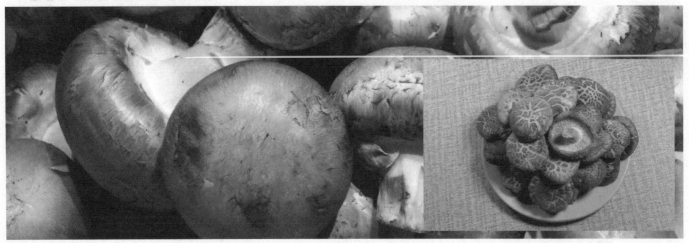

What are Mushrooms?

Mushrooms are a versatile and nutritious addition to a healthy diet. They are a good source of essential nutrients, including copper, which plays a vital role in various physiological processes, such as iron metabolism and the formation of red blood cells. Mushrooms also contain vitamin B2 (riboflavin) and vitamin B5 (pantothenic acid), contributing to energy metabolism and skin health.

Beyond their nutrient content, mushrooms offer unique bioactive compounds with potential health benefits. They are rich in antioxidants and have been associated with anti-inflammatory and immune-boosting properties. Additionally, mushrooms contain ergosterol, a precursor to vitamin D, and their exposure to sunlight can enhance their vitamin D content.

Incorporating a variety of mushrooms into your diet can provide a range of nutrients and contribute to overall well-being, supporting aspects of metabolism, skin health, and immune function.

Top Diseases/Conditions

Mushrooms are identified as a top food for 7 of the Top 100 Diseases and Conditions. However, they were not identified as a Top 10 food for any of those Top 100 Diseases and conditions.

Nutrients?

One serving (84g, 18 Calories) contains:

6 Significant Nutrients	
Nutrient	DRI Per Serving (Daily Recommended Intake)
Copper	29%
Vitamin B2 (Riboflavin)	27%
Vitamin B5 (Pantothenic Acid)	25%
Vitamin B3 (Niacin)	19%
Selenium	14%
Phosphorus	10%

91. Chili Peppers

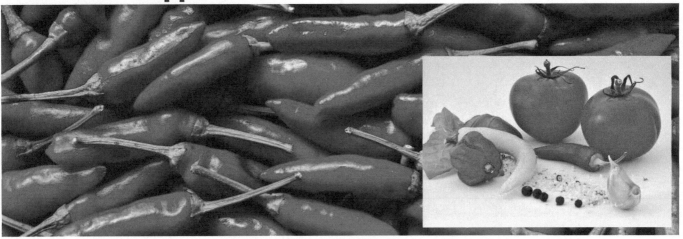

What are Chili Peppers?

Chili peppers are not only known for their fiery flavor but also for the array of health benefits they offer. They are an excellent source of vitamin C, a powerful antioxidant that supports the immune system, helps in collagen synthesis for skin health, and aids in the absorption of iron. The capsaicin compound found in chili peppers contributes to their spiciness and has been associated with various health benefits.

Capsaicin has been studied for its potential to boost metabolism, promote weight loss, and reduce appetite. Additionally, it may have anti-inflammatory and pain-relieving properties, making it a subject of interest in pain management. Chili peppers also contain vitamins A and E, as well as other bioactive compounds that contribute to their overall health-promoting properties.

Incorporating moderate amounts of chili peppers into your diet can add flavor and potentially offer a range of health benefits, thanks to their rich nutrient profile and bioactive compounds.

Top Diseases/Conditions

Chili Peppers are identified as a top food for 5 of the Top 100 Diseases and Conditions. However, they were not identified as a Top 10 food for any of those Top 100 Diseases and conditions.

Nutrients?

One serving (45g, 18 Calories) contains:

| 4 Significant Nutrients ||
Nutrient	DRI Per Serving (Daily Recommended Intake)
Vitamin C	72%
Vitamin B6	15%
Vitamin A	14%
Copper	11%

92. Apricots

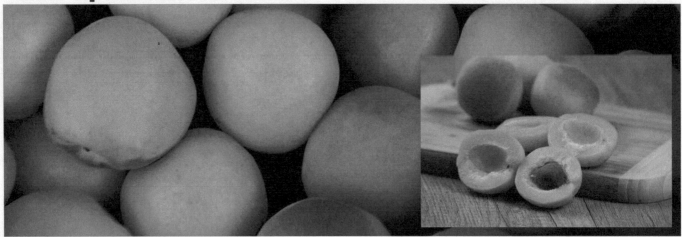

What are Apricots?

Apricots, whether fresh or dried, are a nutritious fruit with a variety of health benefits. They are a rich source of vitamin A, essential for maintaining healthy skin, vision, and immune function. The beta-carotene in apricots is converted to vitamin A in the body, contributing to the overall well-being of these bodily functions.

Dried apricots, in particular, are a convenient and portable snack that retains many of the nutrients found in fresh apricots. They are a good source of dietary fiber, which aids in digestion and helps maintain bowel regularity. The natural sugars in apricots provide a quick energy boost, making them a wholesome alternative to processed snacks.

The presence of antioxidants in apricots, including vitamin A and C, may help protect cells from oxidative stress. Including apricots in your diet can be a tasty way to support your overall health, providing essential nutrients and contributing to your daily fruit intake.

Top Diseases/Conditions

Apricots are identified as a top food for 6 of the Top 100 Diseases and Conditions. Of those, 1 of them rank it between #2 and #10 (Silver Bullets).

1 Silver Bullet	Definition: Top 10 food for each given condition (but not #1)
Genital Herpes	

Nutrients?

One serving (35g Dried, 84 Calories) contains:

5 Significant Nutrients	
Nutrient	DRI Per Serving (Daily Recommended Intake)
Vitamin A	42%
Copper	12%
Potassium	12%
Iron	12%
Vitamin E	10%

93. Oysters

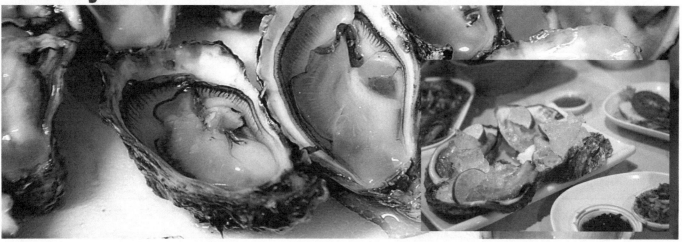

What are Oysters?

Oysters are a nutrient-rich shellfish that offer a plethora of health benefits. They are an excellent source of zinc, a mineral crucial for immune function, wound healing, and DNA synthesis. Additionally, oysters provide high levels of vitamin B12, essential for nerve function and the formation of red blood cells.

Rich in copper, oysters contribute to the production of collagen, iron absorption, and the overall health of connective tissues. Moreover, oysters contain omega-3 fatty acids, including DHA (docosahexaenoic acid) and EPA (eicosapentaenoic acid), which support heart health and cognitive function.

Selenium, another essential mineral found in oysters, acts as an antioxidant, helping to protect cells from damage and supporting the immune system. Including oysters in your diet provides a nutrient-dense option that can contribute to overall well-being, particularly benefiting immune function, cardiovascular health, and neurological health.

Top Diseases/Conditions

Oysters are identified as a top food for 10 of the Top 100 Diseases and Conditions. Of those, 3 of them rank it between #2 and #10 (Silver Bullets).

3 Silver Bullet	Definition: Top 10 food for each given condition (but not #1)
Anemia of Chronic Disease	Hypothyroidism
Cancer: Thyroid	

Nutrients?

One serving (85g, 58 Calories) contains:

14 Significant Nutrients	
Nutrient	DRI Per Serving (Daily Recommended Intake)
Zinc	701%
Vitamin B12	690%
Copper	419%
Omega-3 DHA	99%
Selenium	98%
Omega-3 EPA	91%
Iron	71%
Vitamin D	45%
Phosphorus	16%
Manganese	13%
Sodium	12%
Protein	11%
Choline	10%
Magnesium	10%

94. Cashews

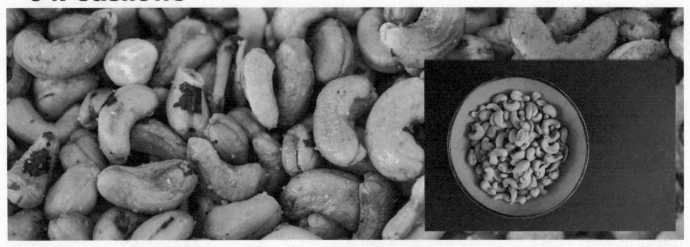

What are Cashews?

Cashews are nutrient-packed nuts that bring a variety of health benefits to the table. They are an excellent source of copper, a trace mineral essential for the formation of red blood cells, energy production, and maintaining a healthy immune system.

While cashews are relatively high in fat, the majority of this fat is monounsaturated and polyunsaturated, which are heart-healthy fats. These fats play a role in supporting cardiovascular health, managing cholesterol levels, and promoting overall well-being.

In addition to copper and healthy fats, cashews provide a good dose of protein, fiber, and various vitamins and minerals. Including cashews in your diet can contribute to satiety, making them a satisfying snack option. Their versatility makes them suitable for both sweet and savory dishes, offering a tasty and nutritious addition to your overall diet.

Top Diseases/Conditions

Cashews are identified as a top food for 5 of the Top 100 Diseases and Conditions. However, they were not identified as a Top 10 food for any of those Top 100 Diseases and conditions.

Nutrients?

One serving (28g, 155 Calories) contains:

9 Significant Nutrients	
Nutrient	DRI Per Serving (Daily Recommended Intake)
Copper	67%
Iron	24%
Phosphorus	24%
Manganese	22%
"Good" Fat	20%
Magnesium	19%
Zinc	15%
Omega 6 LA	13%
Selenium	10%

95. Mangoes

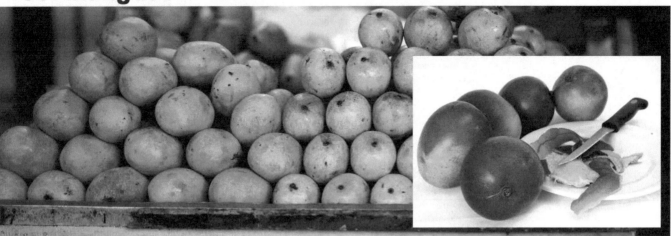

What are Mangoes?

Mangos, known for their delicious taste and vibrant color, are a tropical fruit that packs a nutritional punch. Rich in vitamin A, mangos contribute to maintaining healthy skin, vision, and a robust immune system. The presence of vitamin C in mangos enhances collagen formation, supports immune function, and acts as a potent antioxidant, protecting cells from oxidative stress.

Beyond their vitamin content, mangos are a good source of dietary fiber, promoting digestive health and aiding in weight management. The fruit also contains an array of antioxidants, such as beta-carotene and quercetin, which have anti-inflammatory properties.

Including mangos in your diet adds natural sweetness and a burst of essential nutrients. Whether enjoyed fresh, blended into smoothies, or incorporated into salads, mangos provide a tasty and healthful addition to a balanced eating plan.

Top Diseases/Conditions

Mangoes are identified as a top food for 7 of the Top 100 Diseases and Conditions. Of those, 1 of them rank it between #2 and #10 (Silver Bullets).

1 Silver Bullet	Definition: Top 10 food for each given condition (but not #1)
Genital Herpes	

Nutrients?

One serving (117g, 76 Calories) contains:

4 Significant Nutrients	
Nutrient	DRI Per Serving (Daily Recommended Intake)
Vitamin C	36%
Vitamin A	30%
Copper	16%
Vitamin B6	11%

96. Eggplant

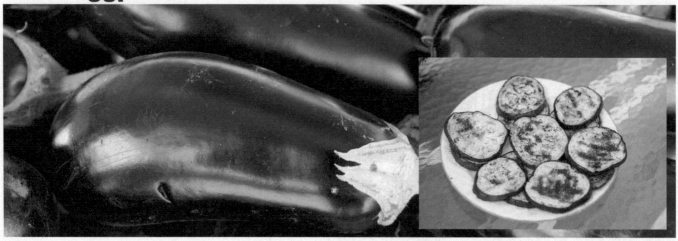

What is Eggplant?

Eggplant, also known as aubergine, is a versatile and nutritious vegetable with a range of health benefits. Low in calories and rich in fiber, eggplant supports digestive health by promoting regular bowel movements and aiding in weight management. Additionally, the fiber content helps regulate blood sugar levels.

Eggplant is a good source of vitamins and minerals, including vitamin C, vitamin K, vitamin B6, and folate. These nutrients contribute to immune function, blood clotting, and the formation of red blood cells. The vegetable also contains potent antioxidants, such as nasunin and chlorogenic acid, which help protect cells from oxidative stress and inflammation.

Incorporating eggplant into your diet, whether grilled, roasted, or included in casseroles, provides a tasty way to enjoy its nutritional benefits and add variety to a balanced eating plan.

Top Diseases/Conditions

Eggplant is identified as a top food for 3 of the Top 100 Diseases and Conditions. Of those, 1 of them rank it between #2 and #10 (Silver Bullets).

1 Silver Bullet	Definition: Top 10 food for each given condition (but not #1)
Irritable Bowel Syndrome	

Nutrients?

One serving (82g, 20 Calories) contains:

1 Significant Nutrient	
Nutrient	DRI Per Serving (Daily Recommended Intake)
Copper	11%

97. Beef Liver

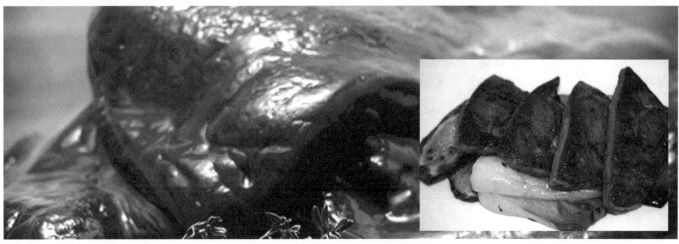

What is Beef Liver?

Beef liver is a nutrient-dense organ meat that offers a spectrum of essential vitamins and minerals vital for overall health. It is exceptionally rich in B-vitamins, including B12, B6, riboflavin, and niacin, which play crucial roles in energy metabolism, red blood cell formation, and nervous system function. The high copper content in beef liver supports the formation of collagen, aids in iron absorption, and contributes to the overall health of connective tissues.

Moreover, beef liver is an excellent source of vitamin A, essential for vision, immune function, and skin health. Selenium and iron found in beef liver further enhance its nutritional profile, supporting antioxidant defense and oxygen transport in the body.

Incorporating moderate amounts of beef liver into a balanced diet provides a concentrated source of these essential nutrients, contributing to overall well-being and nutritional adequacy.

Top Diseases/Conditions

Beef Liver is identified as a top food for 6 of the Top 100 Diseases and Conditions. Of those, 2 of them rank it between #2 and #10 (Silver Bullets).

2 Silver Bullets	Definition: Top 10 food for each given condition (but not #1)
Anemia of Chronic Disease	Iron Deficiency Anemia

Nutrients?

One serving (85g, 115 Calories) contains:

17 Significant Nutrients	
Nutrient	DRI Per Serving *(Daily Recommended Intake)*
Vitamin B12	2100%
Copper	926%
Vitamin A	479%
Vitamin B2 (Riboflavin)	183%
Vitamin B5 (Pantothenic Acid)	122%
Vitamin B7 (Biotin)	103%
Vitamin B6	72%
Vitamin B3 (Niacin)	70%
Vitamin B9 (Folate)	62%
Selenium	61%
Iron	52%
Choline	51%
Phosphorus	47%
Protein	31%
Zinc	31%
Vitamin B1 (Thiamine)	14%
Manganese	11%

98. Amaranth

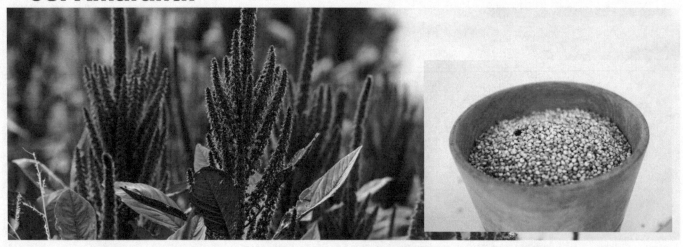

What is Amaranth?

Amaranth is a nutritious, gluten-free pseudocereal that has been cultivated for thousands of years. Rich in manganese, amaranth plays a crucial role in enzyme activation, bone development, and wound healing. Its iron content supports the formation of hemoglobin, aiding in oxygen transport throughout the body, while phosphorus contributes to bone health and energy metabolism.

Being gluten-free, amaranth is an excellent alternative for individuals with gluten sensitivities or celiac disease. This versatile grain offers a complete protein profile, containing all the essential amino acids the body needs. Additionally, amaranth is a good source of fiber, promoting digestive health and providing a feeling of fullness.

Incorporating amaranth into a well-balanced diet adds diversity and valuable nutrients, making it a nutritious choice for those seeking a gluten-free, plant-based protein source with essential minerals.

Top Diseases/Conditions

Amaranth is identified as a top food for 2 of the Top 100 Diseases and Conditions. Of those, 1 Diseases and Conditions rank it as #1 (Golden Bullets), while 1 of them rank it between #2 and #10 (Silver Bullets).

1 Golden Bullet	Definition: #1 Top Food for each given condition (other than Water)
Celiac Disease	

1 Silver Bullet	Definition: Top 10 food for each given condition (but not #1)
Rosacea	

Nutrients?

One serving (1/4 Cup Uncooked, 48g, 178 Calories) contains:

11 Significant Nutrients	
Nutrient	DRI Per Serving (Daily Recommended Intake)
Manganese	69%
Iron	46%
Phosphorus	38%
Magnesium	28%
Copper	28%
Vitamin B6	21%
Selenium	16%
Vitamin B5 (Pantothenic Acid)	14%
Zinc	12%
Protein	12%
Vitamin B9 (Folate)	10%

Typical serving is ½ Cup Cooked, 1/5 Cup Dry

99. Brazil Nuts

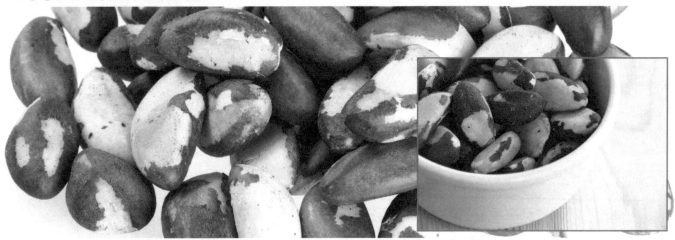

What are Brazil Nuts?

Brazil nuts are nutrient-packed seeds derived from the Bertholletia excelsa tree, native to the Amazon rainforest. Renowned for their high selenium content, just a few Brazil nuts can fulfill the daily recommended intake of this essential mineral. Selenium plays a crucial role in antioxidant defense, supporting immune function and thyroid health.

These nuts are also rich in copper, contributing to the production of red blood cells, collagen formation, and iron absorption. The healthy fat content in Brazil nuts, mainly monounsaturated and polyunsaturated fats, promotes heart health by helping manage cholesterol levels.

In addition to their nutritional benefits, Brazil nuts contain selenium in a form that is easily absorbed by the body. However, it's important to consume them in moderation due to their high selenium content, as excessive intake may lead to selenium toxicity. Including Brazil nuts in a balanced diet can offer a flavorful and nutrient-dense addition.

Top Diseases/Conditions

Brazil Nuts are identified as a top food for 6 of the Top 100 Diseases and Conditions. Of those, 3 Diseases and Conditions rank it as #1 (Golden Bullets).

3 Golden Bullets	Definition: #1 Top Food for each given condition (other than Water)
Cancer: Thyroid	Hypothyroidism
Hyperthyroidism	

Nutrients?

One serving (28g, 184 Calories) contains:

10 Significant Nutrients	
Nutrient	DRI Per Serving *(Daily Recommended Intake)*
Selenium	976%
Copper	56%
Omega 6 LA	34%
Phosphorus	29%
"Good" Fat	29%
Magnesium	25%
Vitamin B1 (Thiamine)	17%
Manganese	13%
Vitamin E	11%
Zinc	10%

100. Pomegranates

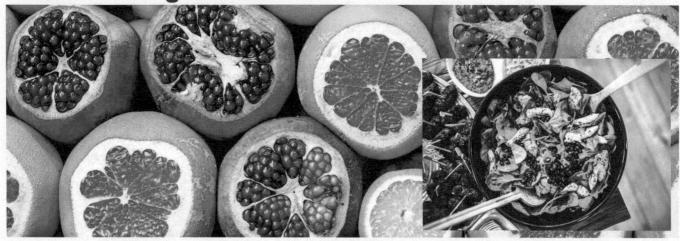

What are Pomegranates?

Pomegranates are nutrient-packed fruits renowned for their juicy arils and potential health benefits. Rich in vitamin C, these crimson gems contribute to immune function, collagen synthesis, and skin health. They also contain vitamin K, supporting bone health and proper blood clotting.

The seeds of the pomegranate are edible and provide a crunchy burst of flavor. Pomegranate juice, derived from the arils, is a concentrated source of antioxidants, particularly punicalagins and anthocyanins, known for their anti-inflammatory properties.

Copper, another essential mineral found in pomegranates, plays a role in maintaining healthy connective tissues and aiding in iron absorption. Regular consumption of pomegranates has been associated with potential cardiovascular benefits, including reduced blood pressure and improved cholesterol levels. Including this vibrant fruit in your diet adds both a delightful taste and a wealth of health-promoting compounds.

Top Diseases/Conditions

Pomegranates are identified as a top food for 5 of the Top 100 Diseases and Conditions. Of those, 1 of them rank it between #2 and #10 (Silver Bullets).

1 Silver Bullet	Definition: Top 10 food for each given condition (but not #1)
Streptococcal Pharyngitis	

Nutrients?

One serving (175g, 145 Calories) contains:

9 Significant Nutrients	
Nutrient	DRI Per Serving (Daily Recommended Intake)
Vitamin K	24%
Copper	22%
Vitamin C	20%
Fiber	19%
Vitamin B1 (Thiamine)	17%
Vitamin B9 (Folate)	17%
Vitamin B6	15%
Potassium	12%
Vitamin B5 (Pantothenic Acid)	12%

"Eat more Fruits and Vegetables" – *Most Doctors*

One of our major frustrations is when a doctor or anyone else advises, "eat more fruits and vegetables." This vague recommendation prompted us to write this book, as it doesn't provide specific guidance. What people really want to know is, "which ones?" To address this, we've created a page that categorizes the foods listed in the Top 100 Foods. This way, you can make informed decisions about which foods to include in your diet.

Fruits

Top 100 Foods Rank	
4	Apples
9	Strawberries
14	Oranges
15	Blueberries
21	Avocados
22	Bananas
23	Lemons
25	Extra Virgin Olive Oil
29	Grapefruit
31	Raspberries
48	Cherries
49	Limes
51	Cantaloupe
58	Pineapple
63	Pears
70	Prunes
71	Kiwi
72	Coconut Oil
73	Grapes
75	Apple Cider Vinegar
77	Cranberries
92	Apricots
95	Mangoes
100	Pomegranates

Grains

Top 100 Foods Rank	
11	Whole Oats
16	Brown Rice
44	Quinoa
59	Whole Wheat
61	Barley
88	Buckwheat
98	Amaranth

Vegetables

Top 100 Foods Rank	
3	Spinach
5	Kale
7	Broccoli
12	Ginger Root
19	Garlic Cloves
20	Carrots
26	Sweet Potatoes
27	Tomatoes
30	Black Beans
34	Lentils
35	Kidney Beans
36	Collard Greens
37	Chickpeas
39	Onions
40	Swiss Chard
47	Bell Peppers
50	Cabbage
54	Squash
55	Sauerkraut
56	Seaweed
57	Potatoes
60	Turmeric Root
62	Brussel Sprouts
64	Beets
65	Cauliflower
69	Peas
74	Lettuce
76	Green Beans
80	Cucumbers
81	Celery
83	Soybeans
84	Mustard Greens
85	Asparagus
87	Turnip Greens
89	Bok Choy
90	Mushrooms
91	Chili Peppers
96	Eggplant

Nuts & Seeds

Top 100 Foods Rank	
10	Almonds
17	Walnuts
32	Flaxseeds
33	Chia Seeds
42	Dark Chocolate
53	Pumpkin Seeds
66	Pistachios
78	Sunflower Seeds
82	Peanuts
94	Cashews
99	Brazil Nuts

Fish

Top 100 Foods Rank	
2	Salmon
6	Mackerel
24	Herring
28	Sardines
68	Tuna
93	Oysters

Dairy

Top 100 Foods Rank	
13	Eggs
18	Greek Yogurt
38	Milk
41	Cheese
67	Kefir

Meat

Top 100 Foods Rank	
8	Chicken
43	Grass-Fed Beef
46	Turkey
97	Beef Liver

CHAPTER 5 – Top 10 Foods By Nutrient

Calcium

Calcium is a mineral most often associated with healthy bones and teeth, although it also plays an important role in blood clotting, helping muscles to contract, and regulating normal heart rhythms and nerve functions. 99% of the body's calcium is stored in bones, and the remaining 1% is found in blood, muscle, and tissues.

Calcium	
Top 10 Foods (of the Top 100)	DRI Per Serving *(Daily Recommended Intake)*
Greek Yogurt	45%
Sardines	32%
Milk	32%
Kefir	30%
Cheese	20%
Soybeans	13%
Turnip Greens	11%
Kale	9%
Amaranth	8%
Almonds	7%

Copper

Copper is an essential nutrient for the body. Together with iron, it enables the body to form red blood cells. It helps maintain healthy bones, blood vessels, nerves, and immune function, and it contributes to iron absorption. Sufficient copper in the diet may help prevent cardiovascular disease and osteoporosis, too.

Copper	
Top 10 Foods (of the Top 100)	DRI Per Serving *(Daily Recommended Intake)*
Beef Liver	926%
Oysters	419%
Cashews	67%
Dark Chocolate	60%
Soybeans	58%
Sunflower Seeds	56%
Brazil Nuts	56%
Pistachios	44%
Walnuts	44%
Pumpkin Seeds	44%

Choline

Choline is an essential nutrient that is naturally present in certain foods. The body can also produce small amounts on its own in the liver, but not enough to meet daily needs. Choline is converted into a neurotransmitter called acetylcholine, which helps muscles to contract, activates pain responses, and plays a role in brain functions of memory and thinking.

Choline	
Top 10 Foods (of the Top 100)	DRI Per Serving *(Daily Recommended Intake)*
Beef Liver	51%
Eggs	26%
Sardines	13%
Chicken	11%
Soybeans	11%
Grass-Fed Beef	10%
Mackerel	10%
Herring	10%
Oysters	10%
Cauliflower	8%

Fiber

Fiber is a type of carbohydrate that the body can't digest. Though most carbohydrates are broken down into sugar molecules called glucose, fiber cannot be broken down into sugar molecules, and instead it passes through the body undigested. Fiber helps regulate the body's use of sugars, helping to keep hunger and blood sugar in check.

Fiber	
Top 10 Foods (of the Top 100)	DRI Per Serving *(Daily Recommended Intake)*
Raspberries	21%
Beets	21%
Soybeans	20%
Barley	20%
Lentils	20%
Peas	19%
Pomegranates	19%
Sauerkraut	18%
Cranberries	17%
Apples	15%

Good Fat

Healthy fats, such as monounsaturated and polyunsaturated fats, are essential components of a balanced diet. Found in foods like avocados, olive oil, and fatty fish, they support heart health, aid in nutrient absorption, and provide sustained energy.

"Good" Fat	
Top 10 Foods (of the Top 100)	DRI Per Serving (Daily Recommended Intake)
Walnuts	36%
Brazil Nuts	29%
Almonds	27%
Sunflower Seeds	27%
Peanuts	25%
Extra Virgin Olive Oil	25%
Pistachios	23%
Pumpkin Seeds	23%
Cashews	20%
Coconut Oil	20%

Magnesium

Magnesium is a nutrient that the body needs to stay healthy. Magnesium is important for many processes in the body, including regulating muscle and nerve function, blood sugar levels, and blood pressure and making protein, bone, and DNA.

Magnesium	
Top 10 Foods (of the Top 100)	DRI Per Serving (Daily Recommended Intake)
Pumpkin Seeds	36%
Amaranth	28%
Soybeans	26%
Brazil Nuts	25%
Sunflower Seeds	22%
Quinoa	20%
Cashews	19%
Buckwheat	19%
Almonds	19%
Whole Oats	19%

Iron

Iron is responsible for carrying oxygen to your muscles and brain. If you do not consume enough iron in your diet, the energy-using efficiency of your body will be affected. Iron helps improve focus and concentration level, reduces irritability, and enhances stamina.

Iron	
Top 10 Foods (of the Top 100)	DRI Per Serving (Daily Recommended Intake)
Soybeans	82%
Oysters	71%
Pumpkin Seeds	53%
Beef Liver	52%
Amaranth	46%
Dark Chocolate	45%
Sauerkraut	44%
Lentils	40%
Turmeric Root	35%
Black Beans	35%

Manganese

It is vital for the human body, but people only need it in small amounts. Manganese contributes to many bodily functions, including the metabolism of amino acids, cholesterol, glucose, and carbohydrates. It also plays a role in bone formation, blood clotting, and reducing inflammation.

Manganese	
Top 10 Foods (of the Top 100)	DRI Per Serving (Daily Recommended Intake)
Whole Oats	94%
Brown Rice	75%
Amaranth	69%
Soybeans	45%
Pineapple	45%
Walnuts	43%
Quinoa	38%
Barley	37%
Raspberries	37%
Beets	36%

Omega-6 LA

Studies show a link between higher linoleic acid intake — the most common omega-6 — and reduced rates of heart attacks and other heart diseases. Some research shows omega-6s may lower cholesterol, keeping your blood vessels clear from build-up that can cause clots and heart problems.

Omega 6 LA	
Top 10 Foods (of the Top 100)	DRI Per Serving *(Daily Recommended Intake)*
Walnuts	63%
Sunflower Seeds	38%
Pumpkin Seeds	34%
Chia Seeds	34%
Brazil Nuts	34%
Soybeans	34%
Peanuts	26%
Pistachios	22%
Almonds	21%
Sardines	18%

Omega-3 DHA

Omega-3 DHA is plentiful in oily fish. Your body can only make a small amount of DHA from other fatty acids, so you need to consume it directly from food or a supplement. Together, DHA and EPA may help reduce inflammation and your risk of chronic diseases, such as heart disease. On its own, DHA supports brain function and eye health.

Omega-3 DHA	
Top 10 Foods (of the Top 100)	DRI Per Serving *(Daily Recommended Intake)*
Mackerel	476%
Salmon	379%
Herring	293%
Tuna	214%
Sardines	173%
Oysters	99%
Eggs	8%
Quinoa	8%
Chicken	7%
Turkey	3%

Omega-3 ALA

ALA (alpha linolenic acid) is essential for good health, but our bodies can't make it, so we need to get it from the foods we eat. It's mainly found in vegetable oils, nuts and seeds. It is one of the 3 main fatty acids: EPA, DHA, and ALA.

Omega-3 ALA	
Top 10 Foods (of the Top 100)	DRI Per Serving *(Daily Recommended Intake)*
Chia Seeds	1097%
Walnuts	159%
Flaxseeds	146%
Soybeans	48%
Sardines	26%
Raspberries	10%
Cheese	9%
Mackerel	8%
Kale	8%
Quinoa	7%

Omega-3 EPA

Eicosapentaenoic acid (EPA) is one of several omega-3 fatty acids. It is found in cold-water fatty fish, such as salmon. It is also found in fish oil supplements, along with docosahexaenoic acid (DHA). Omega-3 fatty acids are part of a healthy diet that helps lower risk of heart disease.

Omega-3 EPA	
Top 10 Foods (of the Top 100)	DRI Per Serving *(Daily Recommended Intake)*
Mackerel	305%
Herring	241%
Sardines	161%
Salmon	109%
Oysters	91%
Tuna	79%
Seaweed	7%
Sunflower Seeds	2%
Eggs	1%
Grass-Fed Beef	0.3%

Phosphorus

The main function of phosphorus is in the formation of bones and teeth. It plays an important role in how the body uses carbohydrates and fats. It is also needed for the body to make protein for the growth, maintenance, and repair of cells and tissues.

Phosphorus	
Top 10 Foods (of the Top 100)	DRI Per Serving *(Daily Recommended Intake)*
Sardines	59%
Greek Yogurt	50%
Pumpkin Seeds	47%
Beef Liver	47%
Soybeans	45%
Amaranth	38%
Milk	36%
Whole Oats	33%
Kefir	33%
Brazil Nuts	29%

Protein

Every cell in the human body contains protein. The basic structure of protein is a chain of amino acids. You need protein in your diet to help your body repair cells and make new ones. Protein is also important for growth and development in children, teens, and pregnant women.

Protein	
Top 10 Foods (of the Top 100)	DRI Per Serving *(Daily Recommended Intake)*
Soybeans	38%
Sardines	37%
Turkey	37%
Tuna	36%
Chicken	35%
Beef Liver	31%
Salmon	30%
Grass-Fed Beef	29%
Mackerel	28%
Herring	27%

Potassium

Potassium is necessary for the normal functioning of all cells. It regulates the heartbeat, ensures proper function of the muscles and nerves, and is vital for synthesizing protein and metabolizing carbohydrates.

Potassium	
Top 10 Foods (of the Top 100)	DRI Per Serving *(Daily Recommended Intake)*
Beets	27%
Soybeans	19%
Potatoes	18%
Greek Yogurt	17%
Cantaloupe	14%
Broccoli	14%
Kiwi	14%
Bananas	13%
Sweet Potatoes	13%
Black Beans	12%

Selenium

Selenium plays an important role in the health of your immune system. This antioxidant helps lower oxidative stress in your body, which reduces inflammation and enhances immunity. Studies have demonstrated that increased blood levels of selenium are associated with enhanced immune response.

Selenium	
Top 10 Foods (of the Top 100)	DRI Per Serving *(Daily Recommended Intake)*
Brazil Nuts	976%
Tuna	101%
Oysters	98%
Sardines	81%
Mackerel	68%
Beef Liver	61%
Salmon	56%
Herring	56%
Turkey	38%
Eggs	32%

Sodium

The human body requires a small amount of sodium to conduct nerve impulses, contract and relax muscles, and maintain the proper balance of water and minerals. It is estimated that we need about 500 mg of sodium daily for these vital functions.

Sodium	
Top 10 Foods (of the Top 100)	DRI Per Serving (Daily Recommended Intake)
Sauerkraut	104%
Sardines	29%
Tuna	21%
Chickpeas	20%
Kidney Beans	18%
Cheese	17%
Beets	15%
Oysters	12%
Greek Yogurt	11%
Milk	9%

Vitamin A

Vitamin A is a fat-soluble vitamin that is naturally present in many foods. Vitamin A is important for normal vision, the immune system, and reproduction. Vitamin A also helps the heart, lungs, kidneys, and other organs work properly.

Vitamin A	
Top 10 Foods (of the Top 100)	DRI Per Serving (Daily Recommended Intake)
Sweet Potatoes	615%
Beef Liver	479%
Carrots	434%
Squash	347%
Kale	343%
Turnip Greens	212%
Cantaloupe	200%
Mustard Greens	196%
Bok Choy	104%
Spinach	94%

Vitamin B1 (Thiamine))

Thiamin (vitamin B-1) helps the body generate energy from nutrients. Also known as thiamine, thiamin is necessary for the growth, development and function of cells. Most people get enough thiamin from the food they eat.

Vitamin B1 (Thiamine)	
Top 10 Foods (of the Top 100)	DRI Per Serving (Daily Recommended Intake)
Green Beans	101%
Peas	33%
Sunflower Seeds	33%
Whole Oats	28%
Barley	24%
Soybeans	19%
Black Beans	17%
Pomegranates	17%
Flaxseeds	17%
Pistachios	17%

Vitamin B2 (Riboflavin)

Riboflavin (also called vitamin B2) is important for the growth, development, and function of the cells in your body. It also helps turn the food you eat into the energy you need.

Vitamin B2 (Riboflavin)	
Top 10 Foods (of the Top 100)	DRI Per Serving (Daily Recommended Intake)
Beef Liver	183%
Greek Yogurt	38%
Kefir	38%
Milk	34%
Soybeans	29%
Mushrooms	27%
Salmon	26%
Mackerel	23%
Eggs	23%
Beets	16%

Vitamin B3 (Niacin)

Niacin, also known as vitamin B3, is an important nutrient. In fact, every part of your body needs it to function properly. As a supplement, niacin may help lower cholesterol, ease arthritis, and boost brain function, among other benefits. However, it can also cause serious side effects if you take large doses.

Vitamin B3 (Niacin)	
Top 10 Foods (of the Top 100)	DRI Per Serving *(Daily Recommended Intake)*
Beef Liver	70%
Chicken	59%
Mackerel	48%
Salmon	42%
Turkey	33%
Tuna	31%
Sardines	28%
Grass-Fed Beef	26%
Peanuts	21%
Mushrooms	19%

Vitamin B6

Vitamin B6 is a vitamin that benefits the central nervous system and metabolism. Its roles include turning food into energy and helping to create neurotransmitters, such as serotonin and dopamine.

Vitamin B6	
Top 10 Foods (of the Top 100)	DRI Per Serving *(Daily Recommended Intake)*
Beef Liver	72%
Salmon	53%
Turkey	39%
Bananas	38%
Chickpeas	38%
Pistachios	38%
Potatoes	34%
Chicken	33%
Sunflower Seeds	31%
Grass-Fed Beef	26%

Vitamin B5 (Pantothenic Acid)

Vitamin B5, also called pantothenic acid, is one of the most important vitamins for human life. It's necessary for making blood cells, and it helps you convert the food you eat into energy. Vitamin B5 is one of eight B vitamins. All B vitamins help you convert the protein, carbohydrates, and fats you eat into energy.

Vitamin B5 (Pantothenic Acid)	
Top 10 Foods (of the Top 100)	DRI Per Serving *(Daily Recommended Intake)*
Beef Liver	122%
Salmon	28%
Greek Yogurt	28%
Mushrooms	25%
Sweet Potatoes	20%
Broccoli	16%
Eggs	16%
Milk	15%
Chicken	14%
Mackerel	14%

Vitamin B7 (Biotin)

Vitamin B7, also called Biotin, 7) is an important part of enzymes in the body that break down substances like fats, and carbohydrates. Biotin deficiency can cause thinning of the hair and a rash on the face.

Vitamin B7 (Biotin)	
Top 10 Foods (of the Top 100)	DRI Per Serving *(Daily Recommended Intake)*
Beef Liver	103%
Eggs	33%
Salmon	17%
Sweet Potatoes	8%
Sunflower Seeds	7%
Almonds	4%
Broccoli	2%
Tuna	2%
Cheese	2%
Spinach	1%

Vitamin B9 (Folate)

Folate (vitamin B-9) is important in red blood cell formation and for healthy cell growth and function. The nutrient is crucial during early pregnancy to reduce the risk of birth defects of the brain and spine.

Vitamin B9 (Folate)	
Top 10 Foods (of the Top 100)	DRI Per Serving (Daily Recommended Intake)
Beets	77%
Beef Liver	62%
Lentils	43%
Turnip Greens	27%
Mustard Greens	26%
Peas	24%
Broccoli	23%
Black Beans	21%
Quinoa	19%
Soybeans	17%

Vitamin B12

Vitamin B12 is a nutrient that helps keep your body's blood and nerve cells healthy and helps make DNA, the genetic material in all of your cells. Vitamin B12 also helps prevent megaloblastic anemia, a blood condition that makes people tired and weak.

Vitamin B12	
Top 10 Foods (of the Top 100)	DRI Per Serving (Daily Recommended Intake)
Beef Liver	2100%
Oysters	690%
Herring	483%
Sardines	316%
Mackerel	308%
Salmon	113%
Grass-Fed Beef	71%
Greek Yogurt	58%
Tuna	42%
Cheese	38%

Vitamin C

Vitamin C, also known as ascorbic acid, is necessary for the growth, development and repair of all body tissues. It's involved in many body functions, including formation of collagen, absorption of iron, the proper functioning of the immune system, wound healing, and the maintenance of cartilage, bones, and teeth.

Vitamin C	
Top 10 Foods (of the Top 100)	DRI Per Serving (Daily Recommended Intake)
Bell Peppers	301%
Kiwi	152%
Broccoli	147%
Strawberries	96%
Oranges	91%
Kale	89%
Brussel Sprouts	83%
Cantaloupe	72%
Chili Peppers	72%
Peas	64%

Vitamin D

Vitamin D has several important functions. Perhaps the most vital are regulating the absorption of calcium and phosphorus and facilitating normal immune system function. Getting enough vitamin D is important for typical growth and development of bones and teeth, as well as improved resistance to certain diseases.

Vitamin D	
Top 10 Foods (of the Top 100)	DRI Per Serving (Daily Recommended Intake)
Herring	231%
Mackerel	51%
Oysters	45%
Sardines	39%
Eggs	3%
Mushrooms	3%
Kefir	2%
Beef Liver	2%

Vitamin E

The body also needs vitamin E to boost its immune system so that it can fight off invading bacteria and viruses. It helps to widen blood vessels and keep blood from clotting within them. In addition, cells use vitamin E to interact with each other and to carry out many important functions.

Vitamin E	
Top 10 Foods (of the Top 100)	DRI Per Serving *(Daily Recommended Intake)*
Sunflower Seeds	62%
Almonds	49%
Peanuts	15%
Kiwi	15%
Extra Virgin Olive Oil	13%
Sardines	11%
Cranberries	11%
Turnip Greens	11%
Brazil Nuts	11%
Apricots	10%

Zinc

Zinc is a trace mineral, meaning that the body only needs small amounts, and yet it is necessary for almost 100 enzymes to carry out vital chemical reactions. It is a major player in the creation of DNA, growth of cells, building proteins, healing damaged tissue, and supporting a healthy immune system.

Zinc	
Top 10 Foods (of the Top 100)	DRI Per Serving *(Daily Recommended Intake)*
Oysters	701%
Grass-Fed Beef	35%
Beef Liver	31%
Greek Yogurt	20%
Pumpkin Seeds	19%
Peas	16%
Whole Oats	16%
Cashews	15%
Soybeans	14%
Sunflower Seeds	13%

Vitamin K

Vitamin K helps to make various proteins that are needed for blood clotting and the building of bones. Prothrombin is a vitamin K-dependent protein directly involved with blood clotting. Osteocalcin is another protein that requires vitamin K to produce healthy bone tissue.

Vitamin K	
Top 10 Foods (of the Top 100)	DRI Per Serving *(Daily Recommended Intake)*
Kale	456%
Swiss Chard	249%
Mustard Greens	232%
Collard Greens	153%
Brussel Sprouts	130%
Broccoli	125%
Spinach	121%
Turnip Greens	115%
Kiwi	50%
Asparagus	32%

APPENDIX 1 – Serving Sizes

In the United States, the Food and Drug Administration (FDA) defines food serving sizes as standard amounts of food that help consumers understand the nutritional content of food products. The FDA establishes standard serving sizes for various food categories based on reference amounts customarily consumed, which reflect typical consumption habits in the U.S. These are not recommendations but are used to standardize nutritional labeling. The serving size on a food label is a standardized measure (like cups, pieces, or grams). The FDA periodically reviews and updates serving sizes to reflect changes in consumption patterns. For example, serving sizes on some labels were increased in 2016 to better match the amounts people typically eat. All nutritional information on the label (calories, fats, sugars, etc.) is based on the serving size. It's important for consumers to note that if they eat more or less than the serving size, the nutritional intake will be different. These serving sizes help standardize food labeling, making it easier for consumers to compare the nutritional value of different foods.

2024 Top 100 Foods Serving Sizes (mg, Raw Edible Portion)

#	Food	mg	#	Food	mg	#	Food	mg	#	Food	mg
1	Water	227	26	Sweet Potatoes	130	51	Cantaloupe	177	76	Green Beans	83
2	Salmon	85	27	Tomatoes	148	52	Green Tea	227	77	Cranberries	140
3	Spinach	30	28	Sardines	85	53	Pumpkin Seeds	28	78	Sunflower Seeds	28
4	Apples	242	29	Grapefruit	154	54	Squash	98	79	Chamomile Tea	227
5	Kale	67	30	Black Beans	97	55	Sauerkraut	236	80	Cucumbers	99
6	Mackerel	85	31	Raspberries	125	56	Seaweed	10	81	Celery	110
7	Broccoli	148	32	Flaxseeds	10	57	Potatoes	148	82	Peanuts	28
8	Chicken	85	33	Chia Seeds	10	58	Pineapple	112	83	Soybeans	128
9	Strawberries	147	34	Lentils	96	59	Whole Wheat	36	84	Mustard Greens	56
10	Almonds	28	35	Kidney Beans	92	60	Turmeric Root	7	85	Asparagus	93
11	Whole Oats	44	36	Collard Greens	36	61	Barley	44	86	Red Wine	142
12	Ginger Root	7	37	Chickpeas	100	62	Brussel Sprouts	88	87	Turnip Greens	55
13	Eggs	55	38	Milk	227	63	Pears	166	88	Buckwheat	32
14	Oranges	154	39	Onions	148	64	Beets	283	89	Bok Choy	70
15	Blueberries	74	40	Swiss Chard	36	65	Cauliflower	99	90	Mushrooms	84
16	Brown Rice	46	41	Cheese	40	66	Pistachios	28	91	Chili Peppers	45
17	Walnuts	28	42	Dark Chocolate	30	67	Kefir	244	92	Apricots	35
18	Greek Yogurt	245	43	Grass-Fed Beef	85	68	Tuna	85	93	Oysters	85
19	Garlic Cloves	3	44	Local Honey	21	69	Peas	145	94	Cashews	28
20	Carrots	78	45	Quinoa	28	70	Prunes	30	95	Mangoes	117
21	Avocados	50	46	Turkey	85	71	Kiwi	148	96	Eggplant	82
22	Bananas	126	47	Bell Peppers	148	72	Coconut Oil	13	97	Beef Liver	85
23	Lemons	58	48	Cherries	140	73	Grapes	126	98	Amaranth	48
24	Herring	85	49	Limes	67	74	Lettuce	89	99	Brazil Nuts	28
25	Extra Virgin Olive Oil	13	50	Cabbage	84	75	Apple Cider Vinegar	14	100	Pomegranates	175

APPENDIX 2 – Dietary Reference Intakes (DRI)

Dietary Reference Intakes (DRIs) are a set of scientifically developed values that describe how much of certain nutrients and energy people should consume. The National Academies of Sciences, Engineering, and Medicine's Food and Nutrition Board issues DRIs, which are specific to the United States and Canada. DRIs are used by health and nutrition professionals to:
- Develop food guides and dietary guidelines
- Ensure foods and supplements contain safe levels of nutrients
- Create educational programs and counseling for consumers and patients
- Assess nutrient intakes and monitor the nutritional health of the population
- Plan and assess diets for healthy people

2024 Dietary Reference Intakes (DRI)

https://ods.od.nih.gov/Health_Information/Dietary_Reference_Intakes.aspx

It turns out that the right amount for any one individual depends on many factors, including their activity level, age, muscle mass, physique goals and current state of health. We chose to take the DRI for men 31-50 for this book, as a benchmark.

Nutrient	Book	Male										Women									
		0-6 mth	7-12 mth	1-3 yrs	4-8 yrs	9-13 yrs	14-18	19-30	31-50	50-70	Over 70	0-6 mth	7-12 mth	1-3 yrs	4-8 yrs	9-13 yrs	14-18	19-30	31-50	50-70	Over 70
Calcium (mg)	1000	200	260	700	1000	1300	1300	1000	1000	1000	1200	200	260	700	1000	1300	1300	1000	1000	1200	1200
Choline (mg)	550	125	150	200	250	375	550	550	550	550	550	125	150	200	250	375	400	425	425	425	425
Copper (ug)	900	200	220	340	440	700	890	900	900	900	900	200	220	340	440	700	890	900	900	900	900
Fiber (g)	38	DNE	DNE	19	25	31	38	38	38	30	30	DNE	DNE	19	25	26	26	25	25	21	21
"Good Fat" (mg)	44	DNE	21	21	28	36	44	48	44	40	40	DNE	21	21	24	32	36	40	36	32	32
Iron (mg)	8	0.27	11	7	10	8	11	8	8	8	8	0.27	11	7	10	8	15	18	18	8	8
Magnesium (mg)	420	30	75	80	130	240	410	400	420	420	420	30	75	80	130	240	360	310	320	320	320
Manganese (mg)	2.3	0	0.6	1.2	1.5	1.9	2.2	2.3	2.3	2.3	2.3	0	0.6	1.2	1.5	1.6	1.6	1.8	1.8	1.8	1.8
Omega-3 ALA (mg)	1600	500	500	700	900	1200	1600	1600	1600	1600	1600	500	500	700	900	1000	1100	1100	1100	1100	1100
Omega-3 DHA (mg)	250	DNE	DNE	DNE	DNE	DNE	DNE	DNE	250	DNE	DNE	DNE	DNE	DNE	DNE	DNE	DNE	DNE	250	DNE	DNE
Omega-3 EPA (mg)	250	DNE	DNE	DNE	DNE	DNE	DNE	DNE	250	DNE	DNE	DNE	DNE	DNE	DNE	DNE	DNE	DNE	250	DNE	DNE
Omega-6 AL (mg)	17000	DNE	DNE	DNE	DNE	DNE	DNE	DNE	17000	DNE	DNE	DNE	DNE	DNE	DNE	DNE	DNE	DNE	12000	DNE	DNE
Phosphorus (mg)	700	100	275	460	500	1250	1250	700	700	700	700	100	275	460	500	1250	1250	700	700	700	700
Potassium	3400	400	860	2000	2300	2500	3000	3400	3400	3400	3400	400	860	2000	2300	2300	2300	2600	2600	2600	2600
Protein (g)	56	5	9.1	13	19	34	56	56	56	56	56	5	9.1	13	19	34	46	46	46	46	46
Selenium (ug)	55	55	55	55	55	55	55	55	55	55	55	55	55	55	55	55	55	55	55	55	55
Sodium (mg)	1500	110	370	1000	1300	1600	2000	1500	1500	1500	1500	110	370	1000	1300	1600	2000	1500	1500	1500	1500
Vitamin A (IU)	3000	1333	1667	1000	1333	2000	3000	3000	3000	3000	3000	1333	1667	1000	1333	2000	2333	2333	2333	2333	2333
Vitamin B1 (Thiamin, mg)	1.2	1.2	1.2	1.2	1.2	1.2	1.2	1.2	1.2	1.2	1.2	1.1	1.1	1.1	1.1	1.1	1.1	1.1	1.1	1.1	1.1
Vitamin B12 (Cobalamin B	2.4	0.4	0.5	0.9	1.2	1.8	2.4	2.4	2.4	2.4	2.4	0.4	0.5	0.9	1.2	1.8	2.4	2.4	2.4	2.4	2.4
Vitamin B2 (Robiflavin, mg	1.3	1.3	1.3	1.3	1.3	1.3	1.3	1.3	1.3	1.3	1.3	1.1	1.1	1.1	1.1	1.1	1.1	1.1	1.1	1.1	1.1
Vitamin B3 (Niacin, mg)	16	16	16	16	16	16	16	16	16	16	16	14	14	14	14	14	14	14	14	14	14
Vitamin B5 (Pantothenic A	5	1.7	1.8	2	3	4	5	5	5	5	5	1.7	1.8	2	3	4	5	5	5	5	5
Vitamin B6 (mg)	1.3	0.1	0.3	0.5	0.6	1	1.3	1.3	1.3	1.7	1.7	0.1	0.3	0.5	0.6	1	1.2	1.3	1.3	1.5	1.5
Vitamin B7 (Biotin, mg)	30	5	6	8	12	20	25	30	30	30	30	5	6	8	12	20	25	30	30	30	30
Vitamin B9 (Folate, ug)	400	65	80	150	200	300	400	400	400	400	400	65	80	150	200	300	400	400	400	400	400
Vitamin C (mg)	90	90	90	90	90	90	90	90	90	90	90	75	75	75	75	75	75	75	75	75	75
Vitamin D (IU)	600	400	400	600	600	600	600	600	600	600	800	400	400	600	600	600	600	600	600	600	800
Vitamin E (mg)	15	15	15	15	15	15	15	15	15	15	15	15	15	15	15	15	15	15	15	15	15
Vitamin K (ug)	120	2	2.5	30	55	60	75	120	120	120	120	2	2.5	30	55	60	75	90	90	90	90
Zinc (mg)	11	2	3	3	5	8	11	11	11	11	11	2	3	3	5	8	9	8	8	8	8

APPENDIX 3 – References

Acta Dermato-Venereologica
Age and Ageing
AIDS
Albany Medical College
Albert Einstein College of Medicine
Alimentary Pharmacology & Therapeutics
Allergology International
Allergy
Allergy and Asthma Proceedings
Allergy, Asthma & Immunology Research
Alzheimer's & Dementia Journal
American Heart Journal
American Journal of Clinical Dermatology
American Journal of Clinical Nutrition
American Journal of Dentistry
American Journal of Gastroenterology
American Journal of Hypertension
American Journal of Kidney Diseases
American Journal of Obstetrics and Gynecology
American Journal of Otolaryngology
American Journal of Psychiatry
American Journal of Respiratory and Critical Care Medicine
Annals of Allergy, Asthma & Immunology
Annals of Family Medicine – Annals of Family Medicine, Inc.
Annals of Gastroenterology
Annals of Internal Medicine – American College of Physicians
Annals of Surgery
Annals of the Rheumatic Diseases
Anne Burnett Marion School of Medicine at TCU
Antiviral Research
Appetite
Archives of Dermatological Research
Archives of Osteoporosis
Arteriosclerosis, Thrombosis, and Vascular Biology (ATVB)
Arthritis & Rheumatology
Arthritis Care & Research
Asthma & Allergy Proceedings
Atherosclerosis
Attention Deficit and Hyperactivity Disorders
Autism Research
Barnes-Jewish Hospital, St. Louis;
Baylor College of Medicine School of Medicine
Behavioral and Brain Functions
Beth Israel Deaconess Medical Center (Boston)
Biological Psychiatry
Bipolar Disorders
BJGP - British Journal of General Practice – Royal College of General Practitioners
BJU International
Bladder Cancer
Blood
BMC Cardiovascular Disorders
BMC Endocrine Disorders
BMC Gastroenterology
BMC Infectious Diseases
BMC Musculoskeletal Disorders
BMC Nephrology
BMC Neurology
BMC Obesity
BMC Oral Health
BMC Pregnancy and Childbirth
BMC Primary Care – BioMed Central
BMC Psychiatry

BMC Public Health
BMC Pulmonary Medicine
BMC Urology
BMC Women's Health
Bone
Bone & Joint Journal
Boonshoft School of Medicine Wright State University
Boston University Aram V. Chobanian & Edward Avedisian School of Medicine
Brain Tumor Research
Breast Cancer Research
Brigham and Women's Hospital
British Journal of Dermatology
British Journal of Nutrition
British Journal of Ophthalmology (BJO)
British Journal of Surgery (BJS)
British Medical Journal (BMJ)
Brody School of Medicine at East Carolina University
CA: A Cancer Journal for Clinicians
Calcified Tissue International
California Northstate University College of Medicine
California University of Science and Medicine - School of Medicine
Cancer Causes & Control
Cancer Epidemiology, Biomarkers & Prevention
Cancer Research
Cardiology in the Young
Cardiovascular Research
Caries Research
Carle Illinois College of Medicine
Case Western Reserve University School of Medicine
Cedars-Sinai Medical Center, Los Angeles;
Centers for Disease Control and Prevention (CDC)
Central Michigan University College of Medicine
Cephalalgia
Charles E. Schmidt College of Medicine at Florida Atlantic University
Charles R. Drew University of Medicine and Science College of Medicine
Chest
Chicago Medical School at Rosalind Franklin University of Medicine and Science
Child Psychiatry & Human Development
Circulation
Circulation Research
Cleveland Clinic
Climacteric
Clinical & Experimental Ophthalmology
Clinical and Experimental Allergy
Clinical and Experimental Dermatology
Clinical and Experimental Ophthalmology
Clinical and Translational Allergy
Clinical Autonomic Research
Clinical Breast Cancer
Clinical Cancer Research
Clinical Cardiology
Clinical Dermatology
Clinical Diabetes and Endocrinology
Clinical Endocrinology
Clinical Gastroenterology and Hepatology
Clinical Infectious Diseases
Clinical Journal of Pain
Clinical Journal of the American Society of Nephrology
Clinical Neurology and Neurosurgery

Clinical Neuropharmacology
Clinical Neurophysiology
Clinical Nutrition
Clinical Obesity
Clinical Ophthalmology
Clinical Psychology Review
Clinical Reviews in Allergy & Immunology
Clinical Rheumatology
ClinicalTrials.gov
Colorectal Disease
Columbia University
Columbia University Vagelos College of Physicians and Surgeons
Congenital Heart Disease
Cooper Medical School of Rowan University
COPD: Journal of Chronic Obstructive Pulmonary Disease
Cosmetics
Creighton University School of Medicine
CUNY School of Medicine
Current Alzheimer Research
Current Opinion in Clinical Nutrition and Metabolic Care
Current Opinion in Endocrinology, Diabetes, and Obesity
Current Opinion in Lipidology
Current Opinion in Neurology
Current Opinion in Psychiatry
Current Opinion in Rheumatology
Current Psychiatry Reports
Dana-Farber Cancer Institute (Boston)
David Geffen School of Medicine at UCLA
Dementia and Geriatric Cognitive Disorders
Dental Materials
Depression and Anxiety
Dermatologic Therapy
Dermatology
Dermatology and Therapy
Developmental Medicine & Child Neurology
Diabetes
Diabetes Care
Diabetes Research and Clinical Practice
Diabetes, Obesity and Metabolism
Diabetologia
Digestive and Liver Disease
Digestive Diseases and Sciences
Diseases of the Colon & Rectum
Donald and Barbara Zucker School of Medicine at Hofstra/Northwell
Drexel University College of Medicine
Duke University Hospital
Duke University School of Medicine
Ear and Hearing
East Tennessee State University James H. Quillen College of Medicine
Eastern Virginia Medical School at Old Dominion University
Emerging Infectious Diseases
Emory University School of Medicine
Endocrine Reviews
Endocrine-Related Cancer
Endometriosis and Pelvic Pain
Epilepsia
Epilepsy & Behavior
Europace
European Archives of Oto-Rhino-Laryngology
European Child & Adolescent Psychiatry

European Heart Journal
European Journal of Cancer
European Journal of Clinical Microbiology & Infectious Diseases
European Journal of Clinical Nutrition
European Journal of Dermatology
European Journal of Endocrinology
European Journal of Gastroenterology & Hepatology
European Journal of Haematology
European Journal of Heart Failure – Wiley, for the Heart Failure Association of the European Society of Cardiology
European Journal of Neurology
European Journal of Oral Sciences
European Journal of Surgery
European Neuropsychopharmacology
European Psychiatry
European Respiratory Journal
European Spine Journal
European Stroke Journal
European Urology
Everyday Health
Eye
Family Medicine – Society of Teachers of Family Medicine (Official Journal)
Fertility and Sterility
Fibromyalgia & Chronic Pain
Florida International University Herbert Wertheim College of Medicine
Florida State University College of Medicine
Food & Function
Food and Chemical Toxicology
Frank H. Netter MD School of Medicine at Quinnipiac University
Frederick P. Whiddon College of Medicine at the University of South Alabama
Frontiers in Neurology
Gastroenterology
Gastrointestinal Endoscopy
Geisel School of Medicine at Dartmouth
Geisinger Commonwealth School of Medicine
George Washington University School of Medicine and Health Sciences
Georgetown University School of Medicine
Gout & Hyperuricemia
Gut
Gynecologic Oncology
Gynecological Endocrinology
Hackensack Meridian School of Medicine
Haematologica
Harvard Medical School
Harvard University
Headache
HealthLine
Hearing Research
Heart
Heart Failure Reviews
Hematology
Hematology/Oncology Clinics of North America
Hepatology
Hernia
Herpes
HIV Medicine
Hormone and Metabolic Research
Houston Methodist Hospital;
Howard University College of Medicine
Human Reproduction
Hypertension
Hypertension Research
Icahn School of Medicine at Mount Sinai

Indiana University School of Medicine
Infection and Immunity
Infection Control & Hospital Epidemiology
Infectious Diseases Society of America (IDSA) Journal
Inflammatory Bowel Diseases
Influenza and Other Respiratory Viruses
Institute for Health Metrics
International Archives of Allergy and Immunology
International Journal of Audiology
International Journal of Cancer
International Journal of Chronic Obstructive Pulmonary Disease
International Journal of Colorectal Disease
International Journal of Dermatology
International Journal of Gastroenterology
International Journal of Gastroenterology and Hepatology
International Journal of Gastroenterology Disorders & Therapy
International Journal of Gynecology & Obstetrics
International Journal of Infectious Diseases
International Journal of Obesity
International Journal of Ophthalmology
International Journal of Oral and Maxillofacial Surgery
International Journal of STD & AIDS
International Journal of Surgery – Lippincott Williams & Wilkins
International Journal of Urology
International Urology and Nephrology
Investigative Ophthalmology & Visual Science (IOVS)
Jacobs School of Medicine and Biomedical Sciences at the University at Buffalo
JAMA Cardiology – American Medical Association
JAMA Internal Medicine
JAMA Oncology – American Medical Association
JAMA Pediatrics – American Medical Association
JAMA Psychiatry – American Medical Association
JAMA Surgery – American Medical Association
John A. Burns School of Medicine University of Hawaii at Manoa
Johns Hopkins University
Journal of Adolescent Health – Elsevier, Official Journal of the Society for Adolescent Health and Medicine
Journal of Affective Disorders
Journal of Allergy and Clinical Immunology
Journal of Alzheimer's Disease
Journal of Anxiety Disorders
Journal of Asthma
Journal of Autism and Developmental Disorders
Journal of Autoimmunity
Journal of Back and Musculoskeletal Rehabilitation
Journal of Bone and Mineral Research
Journal of Cardiac Failure
Journal of Cardiovascular Disease Research
Journal of Cardiovascular Electrophysiology
Journal of Cataract & Refractive Surgery
Journal of Child Psychology and Psychiatry
Journal of Chronic Obstructive Pulmonary Disease
Journal of Clinical Endocrinology & Metabolism
Journal of Clinical Gastroenterology
Journal of Clinical Hypertension
Journal of Clinical Immunology
Journal of Clinical Investigation
Journal of Clinical Medicine
Journal of Clinical Microbiology
Journal of Clinical Neurology
Journal of Clinical Oncology

Journal of Clinical Periodontology
Journal of Clinical Psychiatry
Journal of Clinical Rheumatology
Journal of Clinical Sleep Medicine
Journal of Clinical Virology
Journal of Cosmetic Dermatology
Journal of Crohn's and Colitis
Journal of Dental Research
Journal of Dentistry
Journal of Dermatological Science
Journal of Dermatology
Journal of Diabetes and its Complications
Journal of Diabetes Research
Journal of Dietary Supplements
Journal of Endocrinology and Metabolism
Journal of Endometriosis and Pelvic Pain Disorders
Journal of Endourology
Journal of Gastroenterology
Journal of Gastroenterology and Hepatology
Journal of Gastrointestinal Surgery
Journal of General Virology
Journal of Glaucoma
Journal of Hepatology
Journal of Hypertension
Journal of Immunology
Journal of Infectious Diseases
Journal of Internal Medicine – Wiley, on behalf of the Association for Publication of JIM
Journal of Investigative Dermatology
Journal of Lipid Research
Journal of Medical Virology
Journal of Nephrology
Journal of Neurology, Neurosurgery & Psychiatry (JNNP)
Journal of Neuro-Oncology
Journal of Neurosurgery: Spine
Journal of Nutrition
Journal of Nutritional Biochemistry
Journal of Obesity
Journal of Oral Pathology & Medicine
Journal of Oral Rehabilitation
Journal of Orthopaedic & Sports Physical Therapy (JOSPT)
Journal of Osteoporosis
Journal of Pain
Journal of Parkinson's Disease
Journal of Pediatric Gastroenterology and Nutrition
Journal of Perinatal Medicine
Journal of Periodontology
Journal of Psychiatric Research
Journal of Psychosomatic Obstetrics & Gynecology
Journal of Public Health Dentistry
Journal of Renal Nutrition
Journal of Rheumatology
Journal of Sleep Research
Journal of the Academy of Nutrition and Dietetics
Journal of the American Academy of Audiology
Journal of the American Academy of Child & Adolescent Psychiatry
Journal of the American Academy of Dermatology (JAAD)
Journal of the American Board of Family Medicine – American Board of Family Medicine
Journal of the American College of Cardiology
Journal of the American College of Cardiology (JACC)
Journal of the American College of Nutrition
Journal of the American College of Surgeons – Lippincott Williams & Wilkins, for ACS
Journal of the American Medical Association (JAMA)
Journal of the American Society of Nephrology

Journal of the European Academy of Dermatology and Venereology
Journal of Urology
Journal of Vascular Surgery
Journal of Vascular Surgery – Mosby, for the Society for Vascular Surgery
Journal of Vestibular Research
Journal of Viral Hepatitis
Journal of Virology
Journal of Women's Health
Kaiser Permanente Bernard J. Tyson School of Medicine
Keck School of Medicine of the University of Southern California
Kidney International
Kidney360
Kirk Kerkorian School of Medicine at UNLV
Laryngoscope Investigative Otolaryngology
Leukemia & Lymphoma
Lewis Katz School of Medicine at Temple University
Liver International
Loma Linda University School of Medicine
Louisiana State University School of Medicine in Shreveport
Loyola University Chicago Stritch School of Medicine
LSU Health Sciences Center School of Medicine in New Orleans
Marshall University Joan C. Edwards School of Medicine
Massachusetts General Hospital
Mayo Clinic
McGovern Medical School at The University of Texas Health Science Center at Houston
MD Anderson Cancer Center (Houston)
Medical College of Georgia at Augusta University
Medical College of Wisconsin
Medical University of South Carolina College of Medicine
MedlinePlus
Meharry Medical College School of Medicine
Melanoma Research
Menopause
Mercer University School of Medicine
Metabolism: Clinical and Experimental
Michigan State University College of Human Medicine
Morehouse School of Medicine
Mount Sinai Health System (New York City)
Movement Disorders
Multiple Sclerosis and Related Disorders
Multiple Sclerosis Journal
National Center for Health Statistics (NCHS)
National Institute of Allergy and Infectious Diseases (NIAID)
National Institute of Health
National Library of Medicine
National Organization of Rare Disorders (NORD)
Nature Medicine (since 1995) – Part of the Nature Portfolio, published by Nature Publishing Group.
Nature Microbiology
Nature Reviews Cardiology – Nature Publishing Group
Nature Reviews Clinical Oncology – Nature Publishing Group
Nature Reviews Gastroenterology & Hepatology – Nature Publishing Group
Nature Reviews Microbiology
Nephrology
Nephrology Dialysis Transplantation
Neurobiology of Aging
Neuroepidemiology
Neurological Sciences

Neurology
Neuro-Oncology
Neuro-Otology
Neuropsychology Review
Neuropsychopharmacology
Neurospine
Neurotherapeutics
New England Journal of Medicine (NEJM) (since 1812) – The flagship of the NEJM Group, owned and published by the Massachusetts Medical Society.
New York Medical College
New York-Presbyterian Hospital-Columbia and Cornell, New York City;
North Shore University Hospital at Northwell Health, Manhasset, New York;
Northeast Ohio Medical University College of Medicine
Northwestern Medicine (Chicago)
Northwestern Memorial Hospital
Northwestern University Feinberg School of Medicine
Nova Southeastern University Dr. Kiran C. Patel College of Allopathic Medicine
Nutrients
Nutrition & Metabolism
Nutrition Reviews
Nutrition Studies
Nutrition, Metabolism & Cardiovascular Diseases
Nutritional Neuroscience
Nutritious Life
NYU Grossman School of Medicine
NYU Langone Health System (New York City)
Oakland University William Beaumont School of Medicine
Obesity
Obesity
Obesity
Obesity Reviews
Obstetrics & Gynecology
Ocular Surface
Ophthalmology
Oral Diseases
Oral Health & Preventive Dentistry
Oregon Health & Science University School of Medicine
Osteoarthritis and Cartilage
Osteoporosis International
Otolaryngology–Head and Neck Surgery
Pacing and Clinical Electrophysiology (PACE)
Pain
Pain Medicine
Parkinsonism & Related Disorders
Paul L. Foster School of Medicine Texas Tech University Health Sciences Center
Pediatric Allergy and Immunology
Pediatric Cardiology
Pediatric Dermatology
Pediatric Infectious Disease Journal
Pediatric Obesity
Pediatrics
Pediatrics – American Academy of Pediatrics (Official Journal)
Penn State College of Medicine
PLOS ONE
PLOS Pathogens
Ponce Health Sciences University School of Medicine
Prostate Cancer and Prostatic Diseases
Psoriasis: Targets and Therapy
Psychiatry Research
Psychosomatic Medicine
Public Health Nutrition

PubMed
Raymond and Ruth Perelman School of Medicine at the University of Pennsylvania
Renaissance School of Medicine at Stony Brook University
Reproductive Biology and Endocrinology
Reproductive BioMedicine Online
Reproductive Sciences
Respiratory Medicine
Retrovirology
Rheumatology
Robert Larner, M.D. College of Medicine at the University of Vermont
Rush Medical College of Rush University Medical Center
Rutgers New Jersey Medical School
Rutgers, Robert Wood Johnson Medical School
Saint Louis University School of Medicine
San Juan Bautista School of Medicine
Schizophrenia Bulletin
Seizure: European Journal of Epilepsy
Seminars in Arthritis and Rheumatism
Seminars in Dialysis
Sexually Transmitted Diseases
Sexually Transmitted Infections
Sidney Kimmel Medical College at Thomas Jefferson University
Skin Cancer
Skin Research and Technology
Sleep
Sleep Health
Sleep Medicine Reviews
Southern Illinois University School of Medicine
Spencer Fox Eccles School of Medicine at the University of Utah
Spine
Stanford Health Care-Stanford Hospital, Stanford, California;
Stanford Hospital
Stanford University
Stanford University Medical Center (Palo Alto, Calif.)
Stanford University School of Medicine
State University of New York Upstate Medical University Alan and Marlene Norton College of Medicine
Stroke
SUNY Downstate Health Sciences University College of Medicine
Surgery
Texas A&M University School of Medicine
Texas Tech University Health Sciences Center School of Medicine
The American Journal of Clinical Dermatology
The American Journal of Clinical Nutrition
The American Journal of Gastroenterology
The BMJ - British Medical Journal (since 1840) – Published by BMJ, a wholly owned subsidiary of the British Medical Association.
The British Journal of Dermatology
The International Journal of Tuberculosis and Lung Disease
The Johns Hopkins Hospital
The Journal of Allergy and Clinical Immunology: In Practice
The Journal of Headache and Pain
The Journal of Infectious Diseases
The Journal of Infectious Diseases (JID)
The Journal of Pediatrics – Elsevier
The Lancet
The Lancet Diabetes & Endocrinology
The Lancet Infectious Diseases
The Lancet Neurology

The Lancet Oncology – Elsevier
The Lancet Psychiatry – Elsevier
The Lancet: Child and Adolescent Health – Elsevier
The Mount Sinai Hospital
The New England Journal of Medicine (NEJM)
The Ohio State University College of Medicine
The University of Chicago Medical Center
The University of Texas at Tyler School of Medicine
The University of Texas Health Science Center at San Antonio Joe R. and Teresa Lozano Long School of Medicine
The Warren Alpert Medical School of Brown University
Thomas F. Frist, Jr. College of Medicine at Belmont University
Thorax
Thyroid
Tuberculosis
Tufts University School of Medicine
Tulane University School of Medicine
U.S. Army Medical Research Institute of Infectious Diseases
UC San Diego Health-La Jolla and Hillcrest Hospitals, San Diego;
UCLA Health-Ronald Reagan Medical Center
UCLA Medical Center, Los Angeles;
UCSF Health-UCSF Medical Center, San Francisco;
UCSF Medical Center
Ultrasound in Obstetrics & Gynecology – Wiley; Official Journal of the International Society of Ultrasound in Obstetrics and Gynecology
Uniformed Services University of the Health Sciences, F. Edward Hébert School of Medicine
Universidad Central del Caribe School of Medicine
University Hospitals Cleveland Medical Center
University of Alabama at Birmingham Marnix E. Heersink School of Medicine
University of Arizona College of Medicine - Phoenix
University of Arizona College of Medicine - Tucson
University of Arkansas for Medical Sciences College of Medicine
University of California Health (Oakland)
University of California, Berkeley
University of California, Davis School of Medicine
University of California, Irvine School of Medicine
University of California, Los Angeles
University of California, Riverside School of Medicine
University of California, San Diego School of Medicine
University of California, San Francisco School of Medicine
University of Central Florida College of Medicine

University of Chicago Division of the Biological Sciences, The Pritzker School of Medicine
University of Cincinnati College of Medicine
University of Colorado School of Medicine
University of Connecticut School of Medicine
University of Florida College of Medicine
University of Houston Tilman J. Fertitta Family College of Medicine
University of Illinois College of Medicine
University of Iowa Roy J. and Lucille A. Carver College of Medicine
University of Kansas School of Medicine
University of Kentucky College of Medicine
University of Louisville School of Medicine
University of Maryland School of Medicine
University of Massachusetts T.H. Chan School of Medicine
University of Miami Leonard M. Miller School of Medicine
University of Michigan
University of Michigan Hospital
University of Michigan Medical School
University of Minnesota Medical School
University of Mississippi School of Medicine
University of Missouri-Columbia School of Medicine
University of Missouri-Kansas City School of Medicine
University of Nebraska College of Medicine
University of Nevada, Reno School of Medicine
University of New Mexico School of Medicine
University of North Carolina School of Medicine
University of North Dakota School of Medicine and Health Sciences
University of Oklahoma College of Medicine
University of Pennsylvania
University of Pennsylvania Health System (Philadelphia)
University of Pittsburgh School of Medicine
University of Puerto Rico School of Medicine
University of Rochester School of Medicine and Dentistry
University of South Carolina School of Medicine, Columbia
University of South Carolina School of Medicine, Greenville
University of South Dakota Sanford School of Medicine
University of Tennessee Health Science Center College of Medicine
University of Texas at Austin Dell Medical School
University of Texas Medical Branch John Sealy School of Medicine

University of Texas Rio Grande Valley School of Medicine
University of Texas Southwestern Medical School
University of Texas System (Austin)
University of Toledo College of Medicine and Life Sciences
University of Virginia School of Medicine
University of Washington School of Medicine
University of Wisconsin School of Medicine and Public Health
Urologic Oncology: Seminars and Original Investigations
Urology
USF Health Morsani College of Medicine
UT Southwestern Medical Center, Dallas; and Vaccine
Vanderbilt University Medical Center, Nashville.
Vanderbilt University School of Medicine
Vascular Medicine
Viral Immunology
Virginia Commonwealth University School of Medicine
Virginia Tech Carilion School of Medicine
Virology Journal
Virus Research
Wake Forest University School of Medicine
Washington State University Elson S. Floyd College of Medicine
Washington University in St. Louis School of Medicine
Washington University Medical Center (St. Louis)
Wayne State University School of Medicine
WebMD
Weill Cornell Medicine
West Virginia University School of Medicine
Western Michigan University Homer Stryker M.D. School of Medicine
World Allergy Organization Journal
World Health Organization (WHO)
World Journal of Clinical Infectious Diseases
World Journal of Clinical Oncology
World Journal of Clinical Pediatrics
World Journal of Diabetes
World Journal of Gastroenterology
World Journal of HIV
World Journal of Surgery
World Journal of Surgical Oncology
World Journal of Urology
World Psychiatry
Yale School of Medicine
Yale University

Index

Acknowledgements

We extend our heartfelt gratitude to our Data Science team for their invaluable assistance in writing the code that enabled us to collect and analyze the tens of thousands of studies required for this project. Their dedication was instrumental in our effort to identify the top 100 diseases and conditions, gather relevant studies, and determine our selection of the top 100 foods. Special recognition goes to Matthew T. for his exceptional expertise.

We are deeply grateful to our Statistics team for their meticulous analysis of the data. Their work in filtering duplicates, ensuring the legitimacy of the information, and developing a nonparametric ranking system based on the prevalence of diseases and conditions was crucial to our findings.

Our sincere thanks go to the parents and members of our taekwondo school, Troy Martial Arts. Their constant questions, ideas, and invaluable help with editing greatly contributed to the refinement of this book.

We also wish to express our profound appreciation to our families and friends for their unwavering support and motivation, which were essential in bringing this book to completion, even as the process took longer than anticipated. Special thanks to Tammy T., Martin T., Janice T., Shannon M., Matthew T., Margaret S., and Thomas T., Dr. Lisa B., and Dr. Seifoddin A..

We are grateful to everyone who assisted us in the creation and publication of this book. Special recognition is due to Jennifer M. for her contributions.

Lastly, we extend our heartfelt gratitude to the doctors, universities, hospitals, clinics, students, and journals whose extensive research on diseases and conditions has been instrumental in shaping this book. The insights gained from their numerous published studies have been invaluable in our effort to consolidate and present this information comprehensively.

Made in United States
Troutdale, OR
11/05/2024

24261092R00104